HEALING HEARTS AND MINDS

HEALING HEARTS AND MINDS

A HOLISTIC APPROACH TO COPING WELL WITH CONGENITAL HEART DISEASE

TRACY LIVECCHI, LCSW AND LIZA MORTON, PHD

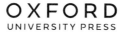

OXFORD
UNIVERSITY PRESS

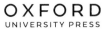

Oxford University Press is a department of the University of Oxford. It furthers
the University's objective of excellence in research, scholarship, and education
by publishing worldwide. Oxford is a registered trade mark of Oxford University
Press in the UK and certain other countries.

Published in the United States of America by Oxford University Press
198 Madison Avenue, New York, NY 10016, United States of America.

Library of Congress Cataloging-in-Publication Data
Names: Livecchi, Tracy, author.
Title: Healing hearts and minds : a holistic approach to coping well with
congenital heart disease / Tracy Livecchi, LCSW & Liza Morton, PhD.
Other titles: Healing hearts and minds
Description: New York, NY : Oxford University Press, [2023] |
Includes bibliographical references and index.
Identifiers: LCCN 2022027333 (print) | LCCN 2022027334 (ebook) |
ISBN 9780197657287 (pb) | ISBN 9780197657300 (epub) | ISBN 9780197657317
Subjects: LCSH: Congenital heart disease—Alternative treatment. |
Holistic medicine.
Classification: LCC RC687 .L58 2023 (print) | LCC RC687 (ebook) |
DDC 616.1/2043—dc23/eng/20220923
LC record available at https://lccn.loc.gov/2022027333
LC ebook record available at https://lccn.loc.gov/2022027334

DOI: 10.1093/oso/9780197657287.001.0001

1 3 5 7 9 8 6 4 2

Printed by Sheridan Books, Inc., United States of America

Photo of Liza Morton by Colin McPherson

For our global congenital heart family; those born into this world with a heart condition, those who love us, and those who heal us

Reviews

"In *Healing Hearts and Minds*, Tracy Livecchi and Liza Morton share a story of courage and hope for those who are living with a congenital heart condition (CHC). The authors through their own experiences give voice to the CHC community. They connect the dots of the disparate knowledge about the impact of CHC. They relate their own heroic experiences as they sought an understanding of how their diagnosis influenced their ability to live a full life. Supplementing their personal experiences are short vignettes of others, who are at times receiving inappropriate medical and mental health support. We learn from their pioneering journey of self-exploration that, even with limited information from the medical community, they sought to understand their feelings and even metabolic resources. The story is optimistic as we learn that with appropriate medical care and a supportive community, individuals with CHC can live full lives, successfully have families, and navigate the complexity of being a successful professional."

—Prof. Stephen Porges, Distinguished University Scientist, Indiana University and Founding Director, Traumatic Stress Research Consortium, Kinsey Institute, United States

"This book is a unique contribution to the world of congenital heart conditions (CHC)—serving both patients and families as well as the clinical care team. Tracy Livecchi and Dr. Liza Morton take the reader on a journey to explore psychological challenges, hopes, disappointments into the new 'normalcy' of CHC patients. The book is motivating, inspiring and helpful. For congenital heart condition patients and providers this book is a must."

—Dr. Dan Halpern, MD, Director, Adult Congenital Heart Disease Program, Associate Professor of Medicine, NYU Grossman School of Medicine and NYU Langone Health

"This is the book for which we've all been waiting. With warmth, respect, and compassion from two highly-regarded authors with lived experiences as well as professional training and expertise, Morton and Livecchi offer an incredible how-to guide for adults everywhere coping with congenital heart conditions. I highly recommend this book for everyone in the congenital heart community—patients, families and health care professionals."

—Dr. Adrienne Kovacs, Clinical and Health Psychologist,
Equilibria Psychological Health, Toronto

"As an adult patient with a congenital heart condition (CHC), I have read many books on the topic. This book, however, provided insights and help beyond so many of the others because both of the authors have CHCs and have personally faced the same challenges that I have. I knew they 'got me.' The unique combination of being patients and healthcare professionals provides the authenticity, credibility, and help that simply cannot be achieved in any other way. What I found most beneficial (and healing) about this book is that the authors recognize the differences between adults who were born in the 50s, 60s, and 70s, and today—and that these differences can be addressed. The authors' insights and desire (and ability) to help clearly come from the heart. Thank you!"

—Rick Puder, CHC lived experience and advocate, United States

"A psychologically illuminating book focused on congenital heart conditions, life-extending recent advances in medicine and surgery, and the associated health and psychological experiences faced by many. The authors write with an uplifting and inspiring sense of courage, optimism, love, and sensitivity, sharing a rich treasure trove of professional psychological knowledge and lived experience. A wonderful, much needed specialist psychology resource to support health and well-being for the congenital heart family around the world."

—Dr. Anne-Marie Doyle, DClinPsy, Consultant Clinical Psychologist,
Adult Congenital Heart Service, Royal Brompton Hospital, London

"This carefully written and touching book takes a novel approach to congenital heart conditions. Written from a lay perspective but underpinned by professional psychotherapy experience and evidence, the reader is guided through their own journey to explore factors that can impact on emotional and mental health and strategies to encourage self-care as well as professional support. The positive effects of storytelling on emotional and mental health for individuals with lifelong conditions and their families are becoming more widely recognized, and this storytelling narrative approach is excellently woven throughout the book using the authors' own stories and those of other adults with CHC, families, and professionals. While it is aimed predominantly at supporting those living with CHC and their families and friends, it provides wisely crafted insight and clear recommendations that all CHC healthcare professionals should be encouraged to read. I loved reading it and will be referring to it again and again."

—Dr. Kerry Gaskin, Associate Professor of Nursing, University of Worcester and Chairperson of the Congenital Cardiac Nurses Association (CCNA), United Kingdom

"Congenital heart disease (CHD) is a physical condition where the heart has developed abnormalities prior to birth. The amazing success in survival is due to the medical advances in making corrections or adjustments to the physical condition. Particularly in adults, while there are physical symptoms, the effect on their lives tends to be much greater from psychological symptoms. These psychological symptoms are very dependent on the individual, what their lives consist of, and how they can cope with them. The future advances in how to live as full and meaningful a life as possible will be the management of coping well, and this book fills a significant gap by offering extensive support, strategies, and techniques to this end."

—Michael Cumper, President of Somerville Heart Foundation, United Kingdom / Lived experience

"This is a book written with kindness and a sense of community. It offers gentle encouragement for people living with congenital heart conditions (CHCs) to validate their own lived experience in a world, and in a body, which may have presented many challenges. The historical background details how medical and surgical advances have increased survival for people with CHCs in the last few decades. The authors explain, with great care, the personal and societal challenges of life as 'pioneering patients.' The expert knowledge of the authors is evident, both in their lived experience of a CHC, and also in their psychological expertise. They use the latter to explain the emotional and psychological impacts of living with a CHC, and they provide evidence-based coping mechanisms. Diversity of experience is recognized and thoughtfully woven together throughout by the inclusion of individual stories. All of this results in a book which will be an important resource for people living with CHC, their families, or anyone working in a healthcare system who wants to take a more psychologically informed approach to care."

—Kylie Barclay, Health Policy Professional, United Kingdom

"This book is a wonderful resource that is greatly needed in the CHC patient and family community. I know it would have helped me at a time in my adult life when I had one medical crisis on top of another. At that time, I reached out for therapy but could not find a therapist who 'got' me. I felt so alone and unheard."

—Paula Miller, Senior Education Manager,
Adult Congenital Heart Association (ACHA), United States

"This book is a fantastic compendium of lived experience and psychological tools that offers practical advice to individuals and families living with congenital heart conditions and the people who are involved in their care. People with congenital heart conditions each have unique experiences. Medical and surgical care has changed and evolved in the last decades, with the individual's expectation moving from survival to quality of life well into adulthood. The timing of this publication is perfect as a tool to support the mental and emotional health of individuals and families living with congenital heart conditions. The lived experiences of the authors, supported by the professional expertise of a counseling psychologist, deliver a compelling read. The personal stories and reflections are powerful in vividly representing the challenges of life with a long-term cardiac condition. While the focus of the book is around congenital heart conditions, I was struck by how translatable the chapters on coping strategies are to all of us, but particularly those with, or who care for individuals with, long-term conditions. The tools for empowerment of the individual in the later chapters are clear and accessible. I would like to thank Liza and Tracy for their passion in delivering this excellent text to advance the healing of hearts and minds. It is a book that I will continue to refer to and share the learning and toolkit of techniques with patients, caregivers, and colleagues."

—Dr. N. L. Walker, Consultant Cardiologist and Clinical Lead of Scottish
Adult Congenital Cardiac Service (SACCS), United Kingdom

"*Healing Hearts and Minds* is informative and thought-provoking in equal measure. The heart is a metaphor for love, for bravery, for empathy, for tenacity across generations and continents alike. So it's perhaps fitting that two people divided by such distance have come together to write a book that holds within it so many universal truths about human existence. 'Patient voice' and 'lived experience' are buzzwords that we hear so often across clinical and support services. Too often, however, this can become more of a tick-box exercise than a reality. This book gently but firmly challenges the simplistic notion that people are 'fixed' when they leave hospital. This is not to deny the incredible developments in medical science that have allowed people a chance of life. Rather, it's an acknowledgment that life and human beings are complex entities, and that we need to treat and support the whole person throughout their entire life. Liza and Tracy have given voice to their experiences and, in doing so, will help to give voice to so many others. Their writing offers a priceless combination of truly lived experience and their own professional expertise. As such, it represents a textbook for us all. For those affected by congenital heart conditions, whether personally or through family members, for clinicians and policymakers committed to providing truly holistic care."

—Dr. James Cant, CEO—Resuscitation Council, United Kingdom

"A book full of compassion and hard-won insight, wisdom, and practical strategies for healing, I sincerely hope this book becomes the classic it deserves to be. While it may focus on congenital heart conditions, there are many other planets of chronic disease that could readily be brought into its orbits of enlightened understanding and gifts of tender self-care."

—Brian Dolan OBE, FFNMRCSI, FRSA, RMN, RGN, Founder of #endpjparalysis, Director, Health Service 360, Honorary Professor of Leadership in Healthcare, University of Salford, United Kingdom

"This book presents a beautifully crafted journey through stories of challenge, adversity, medical procedures, and cardiac events framed by stories of love, perseverance, and hope. The authors draw upon their lived experience of learning to cope and live well with a congenital heart condition (CHC) and their professional mental health training to critically discuss the psychological and emotional impact of growing up with a lifelong condition. This book has important insights and evidence-based strategies for people living with CHCs as well as those who care for and support them. As we become more aware of the need for psychologically informed care and how a child's experiences of medical procedures and healthcare shape care and life going forward, this book is a must read for those interested in adopting a more trauma-informed approach. *Healing Hearts and Minds* is a wonderful achievement."

—Lucy Bray, Professor of Child Health Literacy, Edge Hill University and lead ISupport collaboration, United Kingdom

"In *Healing Hearts and Minds* Liza and Tracy have produced a toolkit for people living with a congenital heart condition (CHC), their loved ones, and the health and social care professionals involved in their care. Their insights gained through lived experience and professional roles have allowed the authors to develop a book that has a unique perspective of the information people with a CHC want and need. As a healthcare professional, this book has helped me to consider how I and those I work with can better support and meet the needs of people with a CHC, going beyond the CHC itself and taking a truly holistic approach to their care. As highlighted in this book, people with a CHC face different challenges than others with acquired heart conditions. Raising awareness of these and helping healthcare professionals recognize these challenges is the first step to addressing them. I'd like to give my sincere thanks to the authors for their dedication to supporting others with a CHC and proving the first toolkit to support the mental health of others with a CHC, for showing them a path already traveled and how to navigate it. I would encourage healthcare professionals involved in the care of people with a CHC to read this book to support their development in the understanding of the psychological needs of people with a CHC. Thank you!"
       —Maggie Simpson, Adult Congenital Heart Disease (ACHD) Specialist
             Nurse, Chair British Adult Congenital Cardiac Nursing Association
                    (BCCNA) and Scottish Heart Failure Nurse Forum (SHFNF)

"Tracy Livecchi and Dr. Liza Morton have created an essential road map to guide congenital heart survivors as they negotiate the lifelong challenges of their condition. Compassionate and wise, it offers the kind of advice that is deeply informed by their own congenital heart disease journey, as well as by their many years caring for the mental health needs of their community. Most impressive is their focus on wellness, which they argue can be achieved even in the face of severe health challenges. The authors offer concrete steps that every patient can take to embrace their lives with their own unique heart."
       —Amy Verstappen, President, Global Alliance for Rheumatic and
                    Congenital Hearts (Global ARCH), United States

"The complexities of mental health issues among patients with congenital heart disease (CHD) are unlike any other. Tracy and Liza are not only well-respected therapists in our community, but as CHD patients, they have thoughtfully conveyed our challenges firsthand. This comprehensive resource for patients, their loved ones, and medical providers is a very informative read!"
       —Lena Morsch, Founder of Zipper Sisters: Women with
                    Congenital Heart Disease (CHD), United States

Contents

Foreword

In contemplating *Healing Hearts and Minds*, we are struck with a remembrance of the epic moral and spiritual journey of the namesake of Sophocles' famed opus, Philoctetes. In briefest and, perhaps, personally biased, synopsis, the renowned master archer Philoctetes sustains unremitting painful wounds, the suffering from which leads to a transformation in his understanding of his sense of worth and value and in his relation with the world about him. It is only when Odysseus allows the isolated Philoctetes to be seen, to have his global pain recognized, and to be redefined by his past knowledge and skills and competencies, that he and civilization are healed and reborn.

Tracy Livecchi and Dr. Liza Morton have harnessed their individualized training and experiences both as mental health professionals as well as adults living with congenital heart conditions (CHCs) to create a first-of-its-kind, easily readable, focused, informative, and entertaining primer and guide to awareness of, and release from, the global suffering that commonly occurs in the setting of a lifelong medical condition. Through personal revelation, definition and explanation, narrative sharing, and exercises, the authors have crafted a framework from which the reader can acknowledge, process, and potentially normalize their physical, social, psychological, and spiritual experiences. In so doing, they define a pathway for redefinition and healing.

It remains a great honor to participate in the guidance and comprehensive lifelong care for young and older adults with CHCs. As care providers, we are given the opportunity to celebrate our patients through their depth of multifaceted challenges and their amazing multidimensional accomplishments. If we practice at our best, we come to recognize early that there is no medical condition that affects only the physicality of a person; to us, we are grateful to Liza and Tracy for their wisdom in calling this out loud, filling a void for the benefit of our patients, their families, and for our colleagues.

Healing Hearts and Minds brings together two individuals who come from different continents, and it underscores that care and caring for those affected by CHC remain global issues. Despite wide social and economic and medical variances for patients and families with CHCs, we witness a core commonality of experience, and we hope that both positive and negative lessons learned are shared between developed and resource-restricted settings and countries.

We celebrate this first joint effort from Tracy and Liza, and we hope that it serves as a platform to see ourselves better, to inform more insightful understanding, and to provide a pathway for more optimal caring and healing for our patients, and for ourselves as care providers.

Dorothy Pearson, Vice President Global Alliance of Rheumatic
and Congenital Hearts, and Former Senior Physician's Assistant,
Boston Adult Congenital Heart Disease Center (BACH)
Dr. Michael Landzberg, Founding Director, Boston Adult Congenital Heart
(BACH) and Pulmonary Hypertension Program, Laurence J. Sloss, MD, Chair
in Cardiology, Associate Professor of Medicine, Harvard Medical School

Preface: Our Hope and Mission

Whether you are someone who has a congenital heart condition, a concerned family member, friend, or healthcare professional, this book was written for you. We understand firsthand how challenging it can be to be born with a congenital heart defect or defects. We also realize that it can be difficult to witness a loved one's (or a patient's) need for cardiac care. Not only are we both mental healthcare providers, but we also happen to be living with our own congenital heart conditions. As "pioneering patients," we have learned to live well, despite our heart conditions, and we'd like to share with you what helped us to do this. Our partnership in creating this book has been a labor of love grounded in our lived experience as patients, having had multiple, often pioneering, surgeries and procedures, but also from our professional training, clinical practice, research, and advocacy experiences.

We know that for many, these defects and any subsequent interventions may create a medical condition, often referred to as congenital heart disease (CHD), requiring the need for specialized, lifelong care. For purposes of this book, we will be referring to all heart defects, as well as the impact they have on the overall function of the heart, as a congenital heart condition (CHC).

What Brought Us Together

Our individual CHC stories are described at the end of this chapter, but we believe that the story of what brought us together is also important. Despite living on different continents and over 3000 miles apart, we have a lot in common. It is our history of feeling alone in our CHC experience that led to finding one another. As is the case for many children with a CHC, neither one of us knew anyone else our age with a heart problem. The only other "heart patients" that we encountered seemed to be decades older and talked about lowering their cholesterol or controlling their blood pressure. For years we each longed to connect with someone "like me."

We remember growing up feeling different at times, overwhelmed by the medical interventions and crises we faced, and confused by the lack of acknowledgment or understanding of the emotional toll. We kept much of this to ourselves so as not to worry our families, always aware of the concern our heart conditions already caused them. Some wider family and friends just didn't get it. How could they without having any shared experiences? Often, even with the best intentions in the world, they either minimized the impact of our conditions or, perhaps worse, looked on with pity or became overprotective. As young adults, we both scoured our local libraries and bookstores for resources to help guide us and give us information on coping. Despite the fact that CHC is the most common birth defect, we were never able to find the resources we needed.

We each separately made a commitment to ourselves to search for answers to better understand our lived experience, and this led us both into a helping profession. As mental health practitioners, it became our individual goal to spread the word within the CHC community about the importance of mental health and psychosocial support. We each knew that there should be more offered to this growing community.

With the development of the Internet, we were able to finally make connections. We were excited at the prospects of meeting others locally, nationally, and ultimately internationally. It was through our individual searches that we found each other. While researching online in preparation to give a talk on body image at a CHC national conference in the United States, Tracy stumbled upon Liza's (and friends') incredible "Scarred for Life" photography exhibition about the hidden population of adults living with CHCs in the United Kingdom.[1] After corresponding around Tracy's request for permission to use some of the images, we both ended up getting so much more. Not only did we find someone else who would understand what each of us had been through, but we both also acknowledged the enormous need for connection, support, and increased resources within this community.

We decided to work together to create the book we had always been looking for but could never find. Who else would be in a better position to do this? At the time of writing, we have still never met in person, but hope to someday! We believe that it is our lived experiences, coupled with our individual mental health training, clinical, and research backgrounds, that make us the perfect team for this very important job. We hope you think so, too.

The CHC community comprises a very diverse group of individuals. There are many different congenital heart conditions which are generally categorized as mild, moderate, and complex. Each of them requires its own recommended treatments and carries its own prognosis. Even for those individuals who share the same age, diagnosis, and medical histories, their outcomes can be very different. Therefore, we have tried to include information for everyone, regardless of where you are in your CHC journey.

While each individual experience varies, there are many similarities. We want you to know that there are others out there, like you, trying to cope and live well despite their CHC. It is our hope to connect you to resources which will help you to feel less isolated and alone. Support is out there, and this book will help you to find it.

Through this book we will share with you what we have learned by drawing from our practice as psychotherapists, researchers, and advocates over the years and most importantly from our real-life experiences of living with our CHCs. We have both experienced many of the challenges that often go along with our CHCs and have, unfortunately, felt the gap in care when it came to considering the emotional and/or psychological effects. We want you to know that psychological and emotional health is a very important piece of your overall medical care. Simply put: your feelings matter and need to be heard and addressed by a member of your healthcare team. Being heard and having your emotions validated are essential to reducing stress and improving the quality of your overall health and life in general.

Throughout the book you will find exercises which will encourage you to reflect on your own individual challenges or goals relating to your heart condition. We encourage you to record your reflections and feelings. Journaling has been found to help in recording experiences, charting progress, processing emotions, and making sense of your experience. We recommend that you find or invest in a journal and keep it near you as you are reading. We are hoping that you will finish this book feeling more equipped and better able to not only survive, but to thrive despite what your CHC confronts you with.

One thing we learned in our work is that every single person with a CHC (and family member) has an important story to tell. As therapists working with this population, we realize these stories are unique and that there are many. For some people, their health story is brief; perhaps they never needed to have surgery, and they did not experience any medical interventions. For others they had surgery when they were infants and have done very well, without any need for follow-up interventions or had no life challenges associated with their CHC. But for many, coming into this world with a "broken heart" can taint their perception of themselves, their relationships, and their worlds. Often it is this group of individuals who must endure the multiple, invasive surgeries and procedures which in some cases are repeated and unexpected throughout their lives.

All too often the emotional and psychological impact of this journey is missed by the focus on test results and physical symptoms. The medical system wasn't expecting many of us to survive as long as we have. For many years there weren't even adult CHC specialists. These caring medical professionals are now trying to catch up with the limited resources and knowledge that they have. Many only recently realized that individuals with CHC have many psychosocial issues that need to be addressed. The CHC community is now starting to understand that this is due to the multitude of unusual and uniquely stressful life experiences many are required to go through, all relating to having this serious lifelong illness. Yet often our care is still "survival" focused, and we are still some way from being offered the more holistic approach we need.

We want to send the message that individuals with a CHC need to have their thoughts, feelings, and fears heard. We want you to know that your emotions are important and need to be validated and addressed. We understand that it can be hard to voice these difficult feelings. Some people worry that they will seem ungrateful for the chance at life they have been given, will appear critical of the care they have or have not received, or don't want to concern their families. If they have the courage to speak up, sometimes they are unintentionally pushed aside, with their concerns forgotten. We suspect that this is because of a lack of awareness or because of unfortunate societal or cultural stigmas which are sometimes still connected with mental health issues. Some individuals have even reported that they wanted or requested professional help but couldn't find it anywhere. Accessing good mental health treatment isn't always easy. In Chapter 10, we will also give some tips on how to find a good therapist.

It is important to know that acknowledging the emotional toll of the challenges that you face does not mean that you are being ungrateful or critical of your care providers or family. It is entirely possible to feel both tremendous gratitude for your life and the care you have received while recognizing the unusual challenges you face and their emotional impact. You are just as entitled as anyone else to have an emotional response to adversity. This does not mean that you are not brave. In fact, it means you are courageous. The word *courage* originates from *cor*, the Latin word for "heart," and it means to speak your truth with all of your heart. If psychological and emotional issues are left unrecognized and unaddressed, not only is it painful, but it can impact your relationships, sense of self, and your overall quality of life and physical health.

It is essential that CHC patients feel as if they can reach out for support if they are sad, scared, anxious, depressed, overwhelmed, or simply emotionally exhausted. We are hoping to increase the awareness of your family members and the professionals who care for you, as well. Sometimes it is a loved one or a healthcare provider who first recognizes the need for mental health support because it is not always apparent to the individual. How a person grew up and what their cultural beliefs are concerning mental health can influence a person's ability to recognize that they may need help. It is our hope that the psychological and emotional impact of living with a serious lifelong heart condition is better accepted, acknowledged, understood, and supported.

Congenital Heart Disease or Congenital Heart Condition?

We want to explain why we have chosen to use the term "congenital heart condition" (CHC) throughout this book rather than the more commonly used term "congenital heart disease" (CHD) that appears in our book title (so you would recognize what the book is about). We have made this decision based on a combination of personal preference and because historically the term "CHD" has been the subject of controversy within our community. Debate reigns as to whether the "D" in CHD stands for "defect," "disease," or "disorder," none of which seem to offer a satisfactory description of living with a heart condition from cradle to grave. Further, the acronym CHD is shared with "coronary heart disease," which implies that our heart disease is something that we have developed or acquired, as opposed to being something we are born with. This misconception often places us into services designed for people with very different medical needs. As a result, follow-up care to appropriate specialists and the need for lifelong cardiac care could be overlooked. As such, after several conversations we have settled with using "congenital heart condition" or "CHC" throughout the book. As a community, we are different from patients with coronary heart disease and we require specialized, lifelong care.

Our Stories

There is no agony like bearing an untold story inside you.

—Zora Neale Hurston[2]

We both have written about our CHC journey in what follows. Both of our stories are filled with strong emotion but also a lot of hope. Each one of us goes into some detail about our CHC and the cardiac treatments we have had to go through. It is important to note that we are both first-generation CHC survivors, and much of our care has been pioneering. Medical care has improved vastly since these early days in many ways. We understand that for some people our stories may be difficult to read. There is a possibility that they could trigger strong emotions in you or possibly be reminiscent of painful memories related to your diagnosis, past treatments, or fears. Please know that we understand if that is the case, and we encourage you to only read the sections of this book that you find helpful. This book is intended to help you to feel more connected and less alone; we want you to be in charge of the information you expose yourself to and believe will be helpful. Simply put: feel free to skip the rest of this chapter if you believe the stories will be too painful to read. All of us must learn what we need to do to protect ourselves emotionally and hold firm to the limits we need to set.

Liza's Story (UK Based)

I was born in Scotland in 1978, with third-degree heart block due to neonatal lupus. My heart beats too slowly to sustain life, which is caused by a problem with the electrical pulses that control its rhythm. I was transferred from our local maternity hospital to Glasgow's Yorkhill Hospital for Sick Children, where I was fitted to an external pacemaker at 4 days old. When this restored life, a cardiac pacemaker was fitted by thoracotomy,

⟩ Thorac Cardiovasc Surg. 1986 Aug;34(4):230-5. doi: 10.1055/s-2007-1020418.

Permanent cardiac pacemaker in infants and children

H K Dasmahapatra, M P Jamieson, G M Brewster, B Doig, J C Pollock

PMID: 2429390   DOI: 10.1055/s-2007-1020418

Abstract

Between October 1970 and November 1984, 26 infants and children aged 11 days to 18 years (mean 5.7 years) received 42 permanent cardiac pacemakers (26 primary implants, 16 re-implants) for congenital or surgically acquired heart block, bradycardia and sinus node dysfunction. Twenty-two patients had unipolar pacing and 4 bipolar pacing. Of 26 primary implantations, 2 had fixed rate epicardial pacing, 16 ventricular demand pacing (13 epicardial, 3 endocardial), 3 epicardial VAT (P-synchronous) pacing and 5 DDD (universal) pacing (4 epicardial, one endocardial). Fourteen patients required a further 19 operations for change of generators (16), ventricular lead (1), generator site (1) and generator encasing (1). Thirty-day hospital mortality was 11.5% (3/26), of which one death was possibly related to pacing failure. Four patients died during the follow-up period (3 months to 10 years; mean 3.4 years). Sixteen of the 19 survivors achieved complete symptomatic relief, without any medical therapy. Our results indicate that modern cardiac pacemaker systems are safe and reliable, and are associated with major relief of symptoms in this age group.

Figure P.1 Medical journal abstract from 1986. Liza is the 11-day-old baby mentioned in this study.[3]

the world's first at the time for an 11-day-old (see Figure P.1; I am the youngest baby reported in the study). I've relied on a pacemaker for every heartbeat since. The first system failed, and it was replaced within 24 hours. I suffered from a stroke, leaving me temporarily paralyzed down the left side of my body between surgeries. My mum was finally able to hold and take me home at 6 weeks old to *love me better*. By the age of 7, I had been fitted with five pacemakers, each by thoracotomy. I remember feeling very poorly and, with broken ribs and a long scar punctuated by a row of thick black stitches, very sore during these episodes in the hospital, my mum barely leaving my side. I focused on getting well enough to be allowed a gentle turn on the ward's rocking horse, which I knew meant it was nearly time to go home. My treatment was experimental, with survival never guaranteed, so while leaving the safety of the children's heart ward always felt exciting, it was also scary. I felt sad for the babies on the ward that never seemed to gain that privilege.

Early pacemakers were set at a fixed rate, so my heart rate could not go up or down. Consequently, I would vomit with exertion or strong emotion and often felt tired and dizzy while my lips and fingers turned blue in the cold. We were told I should be able to function normally which, at odds with my bodily experience, confused me. I remember watching in awe at how active other children were while I was unable to take part in gym lessons, dance classes, or run around the playground. I compensated with drawing, reading, and quiet play. It was hard missing out but more so feeling unwell in an attempt to keep up, and I enjoyed these quieter pursuits.

A kind professor of physics from the University of Glasgow would come to my frequent hospital appointments to teach my much-loved cardiac team how to interrogate the pacemaker. I remember zoning out during countless hours spent lying on a hospital bed, counting the holes in the ceiling tiles, while the team learned how to use a large magnet, and associated technology, to adjust the settings of my device. I felt faint and breathless as they turned my heart rate up and down. My mum always took me to the small toy shop in the hospital afterward for a treat.

At 12 years old, I was fitted with my first variable-rate pacemaker which, although not truly physiologically responsive, enabled me to be much more active. After several cardiac catheterizations, a hole in my heart (atrial septal defect) was fixed via open heart surgery, at 13 years of age. I remember coming round in intensive care still attached to a ventilator and panicking because I couldn't breathe. There were issues with the new pacemaker, which needed to be replaced several times. It seemed utterly relentless, at a pivotal time during my teenage years, impacting the entire family. I started to feel self-conscious about my growing collection of scars. Mostly, my friends and classmates were kind, but sometimes they were mean, and those comments really stuck. Regardless, they had no way of understanding and I had no language to share my experiences. Besides, I hated the pity I evoked when I tried. What happened to me in the hospital stayed in the hospital. I have no idea how my mum coped, as there was no psychological support for us, and having a sister who was constantly in and out of hospital impacted on my older brother, too. I didn't receive any additional support for missed schooling because I was able to catch up by myself and I was doing "well enough." I worked hard, determined to get to university to study psychology. By 17 years old, I was diagnosed with chronic fatigue syndrome and posttraumatic stress disorder (PTSD), but there was no treatment available in the early '90s. It was just another set of symptoms, including nightmares and flashbacks about my hospital experiences, that I had to find a way to manage myself. The smell of toast still takes me back to lying on a hospital bed post-op; for a moment the bleep of a cash register becomes the heart monitor by my bedside; and the smell of antiseptic instantaneously returns me to the surgical theater.

The challenges of living with this condition don't end.[4] Due to the number of surgeries I have had and the amount of hardware left behind, I require specialist pacing intervention, although some nonspecialists fail to understand this and I regularly have to advocate for the care I need. I have experienced countless difficulties with my care since reaching adulthood, particularly during emergency visits and pregnancy. Any "unexplained symptoms" such as the chronic fatigue I have suffered from since my teens have been dismissed as "noncardiac" and ignored. I've learned to manage them by working part time and pacing myself.

Most recently, in 2018, my pacing leads unexpectedly broke for the third time in 7 years. I had to wait for 2 months for a surgical slot for lead extraction and to be fitted with my 11th pacemaker. A month of this period was spent hospitalized, during my son's summer holidays. I felt guilty, having tried my best to minimize the impact of my condition on him. I desperately want him to experience the normal, carefree childhood I didn't have. There is no greater joy than watching him being able to do all the things I couldn't. Navigating parenthood with a CHC has been another challenge I've had to face in the dark, although I am fortunate to have a very supportive husband who is a wonderful dad to our son.

Despite the obstacles, I have always lived as full a life as possible, pursuing the opportunities to make the most of the life I have been gifted. Like many people with a CHC, I am very aware of the fragility of life and determined to make the most of it. I never assumed I would be a mum, wife, aunt, or a psychologist or that I would have the privilege of growing older. I take none of this for granted. From an early age I have appreciated the simple daily joy, wonder, and beauty of life and just feeling well enough to partake. I appreciate how fortunate I am to have been born in a time and place where I have received all of my healthcare for free. I would not have survived otherwise. From an early age I have felt the lack of understanding about the psychological and emotional impact of living with a serious lifelong heart condition and a need to be better understood, validated, and equipped with how to deal with the impact on every area of my life.

Perhaps in a search to understand my experiences, I have always been a keen learner, fortunate to find ways to study and research psychology for most of my adult life. While training as a counseling psychologist, I attended mandatory therapy, which helped me process my traumatic experiences and view myself as a normal person who happened to be born with a heart condition rather than being fundamentally different to my peers. The process of having my story heard, the uniqueness of my experiences and the feelings they evoke finally validated, was truly empowering and liberating. I found my voice.

I now use my voice to promote psychologically informed healthcare for those of us living with a CHC.[5] I often think back to life on my heart ward, to the other children and hospital staff, in many ways my first family. I want better support, understanding, and inclusion for us all.

Tracy's Story (US Based)

I was born in western Massachusetts with dextro-transposition of the great arteries (d–TGA). As an infant, I was suffocating. The two arteries that carry blood from my heart to my lungs and body weren't connected properly; they were reversed. The oxygen-rich blood was sent to my lungs instead of to my body, and the oxygen-poor blood was sent to my body instead of my lungs—thus giving rise to the term "blue baby." My parents were initially told of a brand-new surgery which I might be a candidate for, but that it wasn't recommended as I would "experience a lifetime of surgeries and pain." The doctor recommended "letting her go," and a priest was called into my room to baptize me and perform last rites.

My parents thankfully changed their minds later that night. An ambulance was called and it transported me to Yale New Haven Hospital 2 hours away where a young, second-year fellow had to courageously perform her first atrial septostomy, which was also brand-new, having first been described just 1 year before I was born.[6] This procedure was done to help circulate the blood and keep me alive until I was older and more likely to make it through the complex surgery called the Mustard procedure. This surgery was done in 1969 when I was just 2 years old.

Since that time, there have been many challenges. As a child, I remember feeling ashamed of my multiple scars and embarrassed during physical education class because I often couldn't keep up physically. I had several cardiac catheterizations and then at the age of 12, I had a pacemaker implanted. During those first 2 years with my pacemaker, I required two additional emergency surgeries, which were due to a device and then a lead malfunction. Each of them was extremely difficult for me, both physically and emotionally. During one of those surgeries I woke up and was alert through most of it. I saw blood on the surgeon's gloved hands and felt intense, relentless pain. When I pleaded with the doctor to help with the pain, I was told in an irritated voice to hold still and that it was "almost over" (which it wasn't). Afterward, there was no follow-up or offer for emotional or psychological support for my 13-year-old self. I was desperate to talk about it, but it was never acknowledged as important or relevant to my care. I suffered from nightmares and flashbacks for years after that surgery. Despite participating in individual therapy as a teen, I wasn't diagnosed with PTSD until I was 31 years old.

In my 20s, I was hospitalized more times than I can count. I was cardioverted multiple times for arrhythmias (once just 5 days before my wedding), had additional cardiac catheterizations and two ablations, one of which resulted in an extended stay in the intensive care unit (ICU) for my 30th birthday. My husband and I endured the stress, fear, and decision-making process of getting several conflicting medical opinions about whether or not I could safely get through a pregnancy and the delivery of a child.

Thankfully, I have been pretty stable for the past few years; however, cardiac surgery is and always has been looming in the background. Since the age of 12, I have known I will need my pacemaker changed every 7 years or so (if I'm lucky and the device doesn't fail) for the rest of my life. Over the years I have seen how quickly my cardiac status can change. I know that in a blink of an eye, I could easily be faced with another real-life, sudden nightmare: cardioversion, hospitalization, surgery, or increasing heart failure. The Mustard procedure is no longer performed, as cardiologists have learned that there are just too many long-term issues in patients who have had this type of repair. They now have a new surgery to treat infants born with TGA.

These experiences have shaped who I am today. They have fueled my motivation to support, educate, and above all let individuals with CHCs know they are not alone and that no matter what happens medically, there is always some hope. New technology has saved my life more than once, and that technology is always changing. Despite all of the challenges mentioned here, I have found a way to not only thrive but also to lead a full, happy, and fearless life. It wasn't easy, but I have learned how not to define myself by my medical condition. Instead, I focus on what I can control in my life, and I work toward letting go of what I cannot control. This allows me to rejoice in my roles as a wife, mother, therapist, writer, and friend.

Therapeutic Writing: Your Story

Seriously ill people are wounded not just in body but in voice. They need to become storytellers in order to recover the voices that illness and its treatment often takes away.

—Arthur Frank, *The Wounded Storyteller* (1995)[7]

Writing your story can help you to make sense of it. This has been shown to be therapeutic and provides an opportunity to gain new insights about your experiences. Studies reveal that when people write about the most stressful events in their lives, they experience better health evaluations related to their illness.[8]

We encourage you to write your story and to make notes about your reflections while working through this book. Your story may change as you reflect upon it. New details may emerge which may affect your narrative. We invite you to make reflections about how the content applies to you throughout this book. You could do this by keeping a companion journal, writing in a notebook, or annotating on sticky notes or directly on the pages.

If you want to write down your experiences, it can be understandably emotional. It is important to pace yourself and do this a little at a time. It can be a powerful way to process and make sense of your own journey and feelings. You may feel a range of emotions, and it will be important to take care of yourself. You can use the techniques described later in this book to help you manage any difficult feelings it brings up for you. If you feel overwhelmed, then it is probably time to step away and do something soothing or distracting for a while. It is also completely fine if you don't want to write it down at all. You may prefer to share your experiences in another way, perhaps by speaking to someone or working through them creatively.

Acknowledgments

Thank you to my husband, Craig, my anchor and my sail, who has chosen to walk with me, supporting my dreams, always finding a way to make me laugh; and our wonderful son, Dylan, the child I never dreamt I'd have, who brings joy and hope to every day.

I am also grateful to my mum, Liz, who did her very best to never leave my side as a child during our countless stays in the hospital, always believing in me and finding hope in every situation. Thanks to my brother, Findlay, who paid the price of growing up with an often unwell sister and my late dad, Iain, who shared the gift of lifelong learning. Thanks also to the family, friends, and colleagues who have supported me and visited me in hospital over the years, in particular my godmother, Agnes, my mother-in-law and father-in-law, Lynne and Neil, and my late grandparents, Findlay and Bette.

In debt to Dr. "Bill" Doig, my first "hospital dad," for his gentle approach, the countless healers who've followed, and the National Health Service (NHS), a testament to our collective humanity. —Liza

My gratitude begins with Dr. Natalie DeLeuchtenberg and the many skilled and compassionate healers who followed her relentless and courageous efforts at keeping me safe.

I am beyond grateful for my husband Joe, who courageously fell in love with me and my broken heart. Thank you for all the hand-holding, hospital sleepovers, and for never, ever leaving my side through the uncertain and very scary times. I also hold so much gratitude for my daughters, Sophia and her tremendous advocacy efforts and Grace for her exceptional editing skills. Their love and encouragement keep me looking and moving forward.

And finally, I am indebted to my parents, Alan (deceased) and June, who taught me how to live fearlessly. Their guidance helped me to develop resilience and optimism which enabled me to not only survive but to thrive, despite my lifelong heart condition. —Tracy

We would both also like to acknowledge the many individuals who have helped us to make this book possible. They are as follows:

Oxford University Press and our Editors Dana Bliss and Sarah Ebel

Dr. Michael Landzberg, Founding Director, Boston Adult Congenital Heart (BACH) and Pulmonary Hypertension Program; Laurence J. Sloss, MD, Chair in Cardiology, Associate Professor of Medicine, Harvard Medical School; and Dorothy Pearson, Vice President Global Alliance of Rheumatic and Congenital Hearts, and Former Senior Physician's Assistant, Boston Adult Congenital Heart Disease Center (BACH), for providing the Foreword

Pamela Miner, RN, MN, NP, for generously taking the time to review the medical information in this book

Dr. Dan Jacoby and Dawn Lorentson, LCSW, Yale New Haven Hospital, for providing interviews on living with heart failure

Paula Miller, MSN, Senior Education Manager, Adult Congenital Heart Association, for providing an interview on the importance of specialized care

The Adult Congenital Heart Association, Heart to Heart Peer Mentorship Program, Zipper Sisters, Global ARCH, and the Somerville Heart Foundation, for helping us reach out to the CHC community for the anonymized testimonials and everyone who kindly responded by sharing their experiences with us which helped bring this book to life.

I

A Brief Medical History

Above all else, our collective story of being born with a heart condition is one of hope, perseverance, and the strength of the human spirit. This is a story of surviving and thriving against the odds. It's about overcoming adversity from birth and any, often lifelong, physical limitations, medical interventions, uncertainty, and barriers to social inclusion in order to claim life.

It is also a story about the power of knowledge, science, and medicine to give light and life through countless acts of humanity. Included in this story are the doctors, nurses, and other healthcare professionals saying the right words when they know we are struggling and keeping up to date with and contributing to cutting-edge medical developments while supporting our lifelong healthcare journey.

But perhaps more than this, it is a story of love; it's a story of parents and caregivers who sleep on hospital armchairs when their child is unwell, grandparents who step up to care for siblings, extended family and friends pulling together to visit during hospital stays with treats to brighten the day. It also includes the teachers who provide additional support, colleagues who try to ensure that we are treated fairly, and partners who choose to walk with us along with our children, nieces, and nephews who give us tremendous hope.

If you are an adult with a congenital heart condition (CHC) or family member reading this, we want to acknowledge the expertise, courage, and wisdom you already bring. We aim to build on the ways of enduring strength and coping that you've likely already developed. We know how tough it can be to live with a lifelong heart condition, as detailed in our stories in the Preface. We are also keenly aware of the courage it can take to face the emotional and psychological impact and that even by picking up this book you are displaying an act of bravery. It is very likely that you are already aware of the challenges CHCs can present; however, over the next few chapters we will explore them in more depth with the aim of increasing your insight and understanding of your own personal situation. These challenges described are certainly not applicable to everyone, and they depend on a vast number of factors, including diagnosis, quality of care, age, and general health. We hope you can see this as an opportunity to validate your own lived experience and then in later chapters build on ways of coping and increasing your support system, if needed.

While we tackle the issues that can come with having a CHC, these may not apply to some of you because we each have unique experiences. We understand that there may be some of you who do not want to read these chapters because you think they may not apply to you, or because they may trigger difficult memories and/or feelings. If that is the case, we understand and encourage you to read only what you are comfortable with. We want you to do what works best for you and encourage you to take things at your own pace, skipping any section you find uncomfortable. It may be that you would prefer to begin reading from Chapter 5, where we shift to focusing on developing strategies to cope with the outlined challenges.

These coping strategies may be useful to everyone: individuals with CHCs, as well as their family, friends, and healthcare providers. If you are a healthcare professional working with this population, we appreciate your willingness and openness to build on your expertise and knowledge about the fuller impact of living with a CHC. We also recognize that working with this population can bring its own challenges, and we hope you will also benefit from the coping strategies and techniques.

A Success Story of Modern Medicine: Understanding the Historical Context of Congenital Cardiology

Thanks to enormous medical and surgical advances of the second half of the 20th century, a growing number of us are living with a lifelong heart condition. Babies diagnosed with a CHC today have over a 95% chance of reaching adulthood in developed countries. This figure is in comparison to the much reduced survival rate of 55 years ago, in which only 25% of these infants made it through their first year of life.[1] It is impressive that the number of babies born with a heart condition who survive to adulthood has increased by 70% since the 1940s. For those children who did survive prior to the mid-20th century, life with a heart condition was commonly limited by restricted activity, with "coddling" recommended. For the first time there are now more adults than children living with this condition, and many of us are living well. This is a success story of modern medicine.

There is no doubt that modern medical treatments are transformative, and countless individuals are alive today as a result of this medical progress. Yet we must consider the fuller picture to ensure that while the successes are celebrated, the challenges are also recognized. For those of us born with a heart condition, this medical history is part of our collective story. Understanding this broader context can help us make sense of our individual experiences. In this chapter we consider the historical context of this emerging field and what this can mean for the health and well-being of today's adult survivors.

The rapid development of surgical, anesthetic, pharmacological, interventional, and diagnostic techniques since the 1930s has contributed to this increase in survival for individuals born with a cardiac condition.[2] Arguably, CHC care began with Helen Taussig's pioneering efforts at Johns Hopkins Hospital in Baltimore, Maryland, back in 1930. As the rare female physician of her time, Dr. Taussig was relegated to care for the sick cardiac kids and "blue babies" referred to by her senior colleagues as "hopeless futilities." Her tenacity and drive to solve challenging problems laid bare the building blocks of a new specialty, that of pediatric cardiology and pediatric surgery. After the pioneering efforts of Robert Gross in 1939, who successfully ligated a patent ductus arteriosus in a 7-year-old child, Dr. Taussig teamed up with Alfred Blalock and changed the lives of countless infants by performing the first Blalock Taussig shunt in 1944 in a 15-month-old child with tetralogy of Fallot. This landmark palliative surgery increased oxygenation and allowed the next generation of cyanotic (blue) babies to survive long enough to await a more definitive surgical option that would come in the mid-1950s. One of the pioneers of this surgical revolution was Vivien Thomas, a black man whose place in history made it impossible for him to become a doctor in the 1940s, but he played an integral role as Alfred Blalock's surgical assistant, so much so that the Blalock Taussig shunt was officially renamed the Blalock Thomas Taussig shunt in 2020. The next half-century witnessed extraordinary advances in surgical techniques for specific congenital heart anomalies, although often at considerable risk for those first pioneering patients. John Gibbon was the first surgeon to successfully use an early heart lung machine in 1953, but that effort met with three deaths and only one survivor, an 18-year-old woman who underwent successful closure of an atrial septal defect. This marked an important turning point in surgical options, in that opening the heart to directly repair defects was now a possibility, albeit extremely high risk. The next evolution of cardiopulmonary bypass was extracorporeal circulation by means of "cross circulation" with a relative or donor to support the child's oxygenation during open heart surgery. William Lillehei and his colleagues operated on 45 patients between 1954 and 1955 using this cross circulation technique, with 28 early survivors, with previously irreparable defects like tetralogy of Fallot. The cost of failure in those early open heart surgeries was great, and it involved the risk not only to the patient but also to the parent or the relative providing cross circulation. Lillehei reported a tragic case in 1955 of a mother suffering brain damage during cross circulation for her daughter's open heart surgery, which her daughter did not survive. Another decade would pass before parents were offered better than a 50/50 chance of survival for their child undergoing most types of open heart surgery. This level of mortality risk seems unfathomable today, but it was often the only option for desperate families fighting for the life of their children.

Åke Senning's "Senning procedure" followed by William Mustard's "atrial switch" helped to improve outcomes for infants born with transposition of the great arteries (TGA) in the 1960s. The "Fontan procedure" developed by Francis Fontan in the mid-1970s gave hope to those who otherwise would have faced early mortality with the most complex forms of CHC involving single ventricles, such as tricuspid atresia and hypoplastic left heart syndrome. The "Ross procedure" was first performed in the United Kingdom in 1967 by Donald Ross to improve longevity of tissue aortic valve replacements, with long-term improved survival.[3]

The increasing number of adolescents and adult congenital heart survivors presented a new clinical challenge by the early 1970s: a lack of resources for ongoing cardiac care beyond childhood. Joseph Perloff was one of the first cardiologists to sound the alarm in the United States, presenting

"Pediatric Congenital Cardiac Becomes a Postoperative Adult" at the American Heart Association scientific meeting in 1972 and subsequently publishing this "call to arms" in 1973, setting the stage for a new cardiovascular subspecialty. By the late 1970s Jane Somerville created a dedicated ward for both children and teenagers with CHCs. This evolved into the Grown Up Congenital Heart (GUCH) Clinic at the Royal Brompton in London, and Joseph Perloff founded the first "adult congenital heart disease" clinic in the United States at UCLA in 1980.[4] The formation of dedicated charities to support this growing population of adults occurred in the 1990s with the Somerville Heart Foundation (United Kingdom) and the Adult Congenital Heart Association (United States).

Improvements in anesthesia and X-ray imaging, cardiac catheterization (1940–1950s), the development of the cardiac pacemaker from the late 1950s (thanks to William Chardack, Wilson Greatbatch, and Andrew Gag[5]), cardiac magnetic resonance imaging (MRI), and pharmacological treatments, to name a few, have also contributed to this story of human endeavor.

This story of hope and survival has not been smooth. Behind each step forward lie human stories, often untold, of countless families brought together with innovative medical teams in their dedication to save very unwell children's lives. Along the road there have been tragedies such as Baby Fae,[6] born with hypoplastic left heart syndrome, the recipient of a baboon heart in 1984 who survived for just 21 days post-surgery. These groundbreaking developments, however, have paved the way for heart bypass technology and the possibility of intervening upon almost any form of CHC.[7]

Modern medical procedures can be invasive and painful, and for many children and their families outcomes have been uncertain. Often life for these pioneering children and their families is not easily won; rather it is a tenuous cocktail of hope and fear dependent on experimental medical treatment. If modern congenital cardiology stands on the shoulders of medical giants, it is these families who carry much of the emotional weight of this progress.

With this unprecedented and rapid success come challenges, often unforeseen. While being gifted life, for many people with a CHC, having a heart condition can present many unique life issues from birth which can impact our emotional and psychological well-being. These challenges need to be better addressed in order to enable us to reach our full potential, despite living with a lifelong CHC.

Congenital Heart Conditions: A Very Large and Diverse Group of Individuals

It is astounding to learn that nearly 1% of all babies are born with a heart condition,[8] making this the most common birth defect worldwide. In fact, CHCs account for nearly a third of all congenital birth defects. It is estimated that nearly 12 million people are living with a CHC globally.[9] This includes a wide range of heart anomalies which can vary widely in complexity.[10] We have listed the most common CHCs in Table 1.1 and, for the purpose of simplicity, we have provided a brief explanation of each condition. The heart is a complex organ; for a fuller, more comprehensive description please consult a medical source or discuss with your healthcare provider.[11]

Perhaps more than any other organ in the body, the heart carries a cultural significance. Back in the 4th century BCE, the Greek philosopher Aristotle proposed that the human heart was the center of intelligence, while 600 years later the Greek physician Galen theorized it was the soul. By 1628 the English physician William Harvey described the heart as a mechanical pump circulating blood around the body. Yet a metaphysical understanding of the heart persists to this day: we still get to "the heart of the matter," love is "heartfelt," when we suffer loss we are left "heartbroken," while the strong and brave possess "the heart of a lion."

Simply put, the function of the heart is fundamental to a healthy life as it is responsible for oxygenating our bodies. A structurally correct heart will have four hollow chambers, two on the right side and two on the left side. The right side moves the blood to the lungs through our pulmonary arteries. In the lungs the blood becomes oxygenated and then the pulmonary veins bring it to the left side of the heart. The left side of the heart then delivers the freshly oxygenated blood to the rest of the body through the aorta. In someone with a CHC, the structure of their heart is formed differently during pregnancy. CHCs develop in utero, usually during the first 6 weeks, which is when the heart and major blood vessels develop. The heart is an electrical organ that beats in a steady rhythm determined by how much oxygen is required by the body. This is controlled by the autonomic nervous system. For some people with a CHC the conduction of this electrical signal through the heart is problematic (e.g., heart block) from birth,

Table 1.1 Common Congenital Heart Conditions (CHCs)

Congenital Heart Condition	Prevalence and Percentages of Congenital Heart Condition Subtype	Brief Description of Condition
Ventricular septal defect (VSD)	35.56%	A hole between the two chambers in the lower part of the heart (ventricles)
Atrial septal defect (ASD)	15.378%	A hole between the two chambers in the upper part of the heart (atrium)
Patent ductus arteriosus	10.172%	A fetal vessel connecting the aorta to the pulmonary artery that doesn't close at birth
Pulmonary stenosis	6.233%	When the pulmonary valve is too small, narrow, or stiff
Tetralogy of Fallot	4.422%	A combination of ventricular septal defect and pulmonary stenosis
Transposition of the great arteries (TGA)	3.819%	The aorta and pulmonary arteries are reversed
Atrioventricular septal defect	3.595%	A VSD and ASD that affects the valves between the upper and lower chambers
Coarctation of the aorta	3.570%	There is narrowing of the aorta
Pulmonary arteriovenous aneurysm fistula or malformation	2.975%	Abnormal connection between pulmonary artery and pulmonary vein
Congenital heart block	3.223%	The electrical signal between the top and bottom chambers is blocked, meaning the heart rate is too slow (can be varying degrees from first to third/complete degree heart block)
Aortic valve insufficiency	2.318%	The aortic valve doesn't close tightly, causing the blood to flow backward
Aortic stenosis	2.334%	The aortic valve is too small, narrow, or stiff
Hypoplastic left heart syndrome (HLHS)	2.564%	The left side of the heart (aorta, aortic and mitral valves, left ventricle) is underdeveloped and does not function properly
Mitral insufficiency	1.348%	The mitral valve doesn't close tightly, causing the blood to flow backward into your heart
Tricuspid atresia or stenosis	1.071%	When the tricuspid valve does not develop properly

while others with a CHC may acquire electrical problems following surgical procedures.

Understandably, many people want to know what caused their CHC.
The evidence suggests that genetic abnormalities from either parent
can contribute to increased risk for some heart defects such as hypoplastic left heart syndrome and tetralogy of Fallot. Other risk factors for
CHC include certain maternal illnesses such as rubella, lupus (which
specifically can contribute to congenital heart block), and fetal alcohol
syndrome. Certain medications (e.g., lithium) taken by the mother and
environmental toxins can also increase risk of CHCs. The exact cause of
most CHCs is often unknown and likely results from an accumulation
of risk factors,[12] although there is a lot of ongoing research to better
understand this.[13] CHC conditions are also more common in certain
genetic conditions such as Down syndrome, DiGeorge syndrome, and
Williams syndrome, although in this book we will focus specifically
on CHCs.

Despite being the most common birth defect, there isn't a lot of education and outreach done as compared to some other health conditions. For
instance, a CHC occurs in approximately 1 in 110 births, compared to new
childhood cancer diagnoses, which are made in 1 of every 6024 children
and teens annually.[14] This lack of public awareness can make it more difficult for individuals to know that there are others like them and to find the
care and support that they need. This is just one reason why raising awareness and advocacy is so important.

For those individuals who are able to make a connection with someone
else with the same condition, many report how surprised they are to find
how unique each of these CHCs is and how different patient outcomes can
be, even with the same diagnosis, age, and medical history. Some people
find these conversations extremely rewarding and satisfying, and some even
build lifelong friendships with one another. Others find the meetings unsettling, and some feel sad or scared, particularly if the other individual isn't
doing as well physically as they are, or vice versa. Some individuals have also
shared their surprise when meeting another individual with a similar diagnosis and hearing about different choices that were made in terms of their
treatment and lifestyle. If you have the opportunity to meet another person
with a CHC, we recommend that you keep this wide range of perspectives
and outcomes in mind.

There are many different factors that can contribute to our symptoms, recommended medical interventions, and overall quality of life. For some individuals with "simple" CHCs, they may never have needed surgical intervention, or perhaps they had one surgery as a baby and do not need any additional treatment. For them, their journey is smoother: they may be able to, for the most part, forget about their condition and live a "normal life."

For others with more "moderate" and "complex" diagnoses, there is a huge range in the number of procedures, surgeries, and hospitalizations we may have experienced. Since there is almost no medical cure for CHC, some of us must learn to live with a serious, ongoing health condition. Some of us face exposure to a number of unique and abrupt cardiac events, which can cause a loss of control, feelings of helplessness, and exposure to potentially traumatic medical procedures. Those procedures may include pacemaker implant, implantable cardioverter-defibrillator (ICD) shock, and cardiac surgery.[15] We might also have to endure emergency trips to the hospital; unanticipated, uncomfortable physical symptoms; and/or uncertain diagnoses. For some of us, living with a CHC can at times feel relentless. The emotional aspect can be further complicated for some by the knowledge of needing future cardiac surgeries, procedures, a lifetime of medical monitoring and concerns about decline in health, and the possible need for a transplant.

It isn't just our conditions that differ. These medical events may have occurred at quite different times in our lives, thereby having a different impact, for example, on our education, relationships, and life choices. To illustrate, for individuals with dextro-transposition of the great arteries (d-TGA), there are three different surgeries that they could have had, depending on the year they were born and the center that treated them. Their medical future can look very different depending on which surgery they ended up having, at what age it was performed, and a number of other variables such as other health issues, medical complications, access to medical care, and quality of ongoing follow-up care.

Holly asked her adult congenital heart disease (ACHD) specialist to connect her with another adult who had a similar diagnosis. She had never met another person with a CHC and was thrilled to be introduced to another woman who was the same age and had the exact same surgical history. However, she was very surprised when she found out that this individual was much less symptomatic, was able to tolerate a lot more physical activity, and had never been prescribed medication, which she had been on for years. While she was happy for her new peer connection, she was also left feeling confused about the extreme differences in their overall cardiac ability and lifestyle.

Further, we each have different life circumstances that impact how our medical condition was handled within the family and experiences with our peers, educators, and friends. Our CHC is only a part of us, and each of us brings a wide range of personalities, attributes, strengths, and vulnerabilities. In short, every one of us has a unique story. While it can be helpful to share commonalities, it is important to keep these diverse experiences in mind when you are hearing about and sharing your story with others.

The Road Less Traveled: Living with a Lifelong Medical Condition

Unless you live with congenital heart defects, it's very difficult to fully appreciate the challenges they bring.

—Zeb, 55 years old, United Kingdom

Unlike most acquired health problems, we are born with this condition; our CHC is there from the start, and we simply do not know life without it (although it is important to note that some people are not diagnosed until adulthood). As such, it can become part of our identity—shaping our relationship with our body, others, and our world, in both positive and negative ways.

We learn to overcome adversity from birth by honing personal strength, resilience, and determination. We grow up with an understanding of how precious life is, and we learn to make the very best of it, to take one step at a time, to value those who are important to us, and to focus on what we can do. Many of us are humbled by our reliance on others during times of poor health, fostering empathy for "underdogs" often drawn into helping professions or other efforts to create meaning and contribute to society.

At the same time, we may sense from an early age that others see us differently, that something about us can evoke anxiety and distress in our parents, caregivers, and others. Most of us just want to be seen as a normal person who just happens to have been born with a cardiac condition, which of course we are, but often we learn early on that our CHC can mark us as different, and we may face discrimination. Sometimes this results in us learning to hide or reject this part of ourselves to gain social acceptance, to avoid pity, or to avoid raising concern. Since a CHC is often an "invisible condition," this can be easy to do but at the cost of being unable to be your "true self." Some people with a CHC describe "coming out" in adulthood by becoming more open about their condition, finding their voice, and learning to seek acceptance and support. Indeed, there is growing evidence to suggest that being proud of your condition by "owning it" and embracing self-management leads to improved psychological health, and we will discuss this more in Chapter 10.

Our experience of childhood may have been less carefree and different from our peers. We may have been very aware of our own mortality and experienced and witnessed suffering from infancy. Our CHC can create obstacles that we must learn to navigate around from birth. Many of us live through more challenges in childhood alone than most people will face in a lifetime. Some of us miss out on aspects of life that our peers can take for granted, and we lack the social network to share our lived experience with others. Proactively reaching out to ensure we develop a social network full of people that we trust, enjoy, and feel safe expressing ourselves with can help to protect our mental health, and we will discuss this more in Chapter 8.

It has also been found that people with CHCs are at greater risk of neurocognitive difficulties, including attention-deficit/hyperactivity disorder (ADHD),[16] which can negatively impact quality of life. We know that a large proportion of infants with a CHC experience problems with feeding,[17] sleeping, settling, soothing, and autonomic and motor organization, which can impact on early attachment with the main caregiver. Having a CHC can also put you at higher risk of a low-level developmental delay, including cognitive, attention, and executive functioning difficulties, and problems with motor and language skills.[18] These neurocognitive difficulties are only recently being recognized and often go undetected, potentially having a negative impact on self-esteem, education, and employment throughout life. It is important they are assessed by a healthcare professional to enable appropriate support. If you suspect this is an issue that has been holding you back, we recommend you raise it with your care team and seek a referral to a qualified professional.

Growing Up as a Miracle Baby

Some early CHC survivors were told by their cardiologists at a young age that they were "cured" or that nonspecialist cardiac follow-up was adequate. In fact, for some time this was believed to be the case. We may have been reassured that our childhood surgery had corrected our heart condition and that no follow-up was needed. A large percentage of this group of individuals can end up "lost" because they have not obtained the cardiac follow-up and care that is needed.

Unfortunately, many such individuals, after years of clinical stability, experience deterioration in their health and ability to function.[19] Understandably, these individuals may feel shocked, angry, frightened, and overwhelmed. This return of symptoms can propel the individual to recount previous hospitalizations which may only contribute to their anxiety, fear, and uncertainty about their future.[20] It is vital they are able to access the appropriate care and support they need.

If you are an individual under the care of a "non-CHC" healthcare provider, we strongly recommend that you ask for a referral to see a cardiologist who specializes in adult CHCs, even if you are doing well physically. Sometimes just having one evaluation is enough to ensure that you are getting the right type of care and follow-up. If you are a non-CHC provider reading this, we applaud you in your efforts to help this patient population and urge you to refer any individuals with CHC that you encounter for an evaluation at an ACHD center.

Those of us born between the 1940s and the 1980s are often considered first- (and second-) generation CHC "pioneering patients" (although most CHC survivors are in many ways pioneers because we are such a medically new population). For those of us who have undergone pioneering medical care, our prognosis may have been uncertain. While we were the "lucky ones" who benefited from brand-new medical technology and surgical advances, being dependent on novel, lifelong medical care can, in itself, present unique additional challenges.[21]

For example, early pacemakers in the 1950s comprised large external units which exerted a 50- to 150-volt charge to the body, causing pain, blisters, and limiting mobility (the child had to be attached to the unit). In the late 1950s, pacing leads were developed that could be placed directly onto the heart, enabling the use of a much smaller voltage. However, this involved more invasive surgery while the external "battery" unit had to be plugged into the wall, limiting movement. In the 1960s the "wearable" pacemaker was invented with a smaller external battery unit that could be carried around by the child. The 1970s brought a small battery that could be fitted inside the body, designed for longer-term use. These early devices were set at a fixed rate, meaning that the device overrode the natural physiology of the body and the child's heart rate could not go up or down, limiting physical exertion. Early devices (even fully implantable ones) were put into clinical use immediately, with any faults being corrected based on clinical experiences, because most of the early patients were close to death, and no other treatments existed.[22] Device and lead failures were common in these early prototypes,[23] while the psychological impact of depending on this experimental, novel, and invasive technology was barely recognized. With the rise of the computer age, today's pacemakers are significantly more reliable and sophisticated, but it is important to understand how far we have come in only a generation or two to fully appreciate the lived experience of early survivors.

Throughout our lives we may have lived with medical uncertainty and been told by our care team that "We don't know what your prognosis is" or "You are one of the first to have had this surgery, procedure, medicine, or device." Our care team and their medical students may have learned from and on us, perhaps gathering at the foot of our hospital bed to discuss our case in the third person. While medical teaching is important, even with the very best intentions, this may have left us feeling, at times, like a "medical novelty" or "guinea pig." We may have felt the uncertainty and concern our presentation evoked in our medical team and families, concluding that we should suppress our own feelings to protect them and not "add to the burden." Often we develop a "dark humor" to ease the tension or denial as a defense. While these may be useful coping strategies, and help us develop a great sense of humor, they can mask deeper concerns.

In the early days, little consideration was given to the emotional and psychological impact of living with a serious medical condition, partly because this knowledge was just not available and care was "survival focused." Even young children were rewarded for being a "good patient" for keeping quiet and still, often being rewarded with a sticker for such behavior which was labeled as "bravery." While being quiet and still is perhaps necessary for some procedures, if we are unable to express a normal response to pain and distress, even after the procedure, we can learn to suppress our feelings and needs.[24] The truth is that expressing our feelings and vulnerability is also brave, but this is something that some of us have to learn to do, in a healthy way, as adults (see Chapters 5–9).

Being dependent on experimental treatment can involve exposure to invasive medical procedures such as X-rays, echocardiograms, pacemaker interrogations, and blood tests as outcomes are closely monitored which can be distressing, daunting, and difficult to make sense of for a child. Further, physically restraining children for clinical procedures was and is still common practice, adding to feelings of disempowerment and impacting on feelings of trust. Often the primary caregiver is asked to assist with restraint, which can be distressing for both parent and child. Evidence suggests that holding or restraining a child against their wishes for a procedure results in children experiencing short- and long-term distress, a loss of trust with health professionals and services, and future procedural anxiety. Thankfully there are ongoing efforts to develop international rights–based standards to guide clinical holding of children during medical procedures which aim to address these concerns and improve care.[25]

Prior to the 1980s cardiac surgery was exploratory, and adequate anesthesia was not always used on babies and some children, due to limitations in anesthetic care and a mistaken belief that they could not feel pain. Studies suggest if pain is not adequately managed, individuals may become hypersensitive to pain and more susceptible to psychosomatic symptoms in adulthood.[26] While understanding of pain in neonates has vastly improved over the last several decades, this may be relevant to early survivors.

In the early days, it was not uncommon for children to be separated from their main caregivers in the hospital and in intensive care, and during medical procedures and surgery with restricted visiting. Some early CHC survivors recall being hospitalized for 6 months or more, recovering from cardiac surgery, in an "oxygen tent" with occasional visits from family. Others recall being taken away from their parents for surgery and waking in the recovery room to their absence. As such, this early separation, during early traumatic situations, may have a lasting impact on many individuals who are now adults (we will go into this in more detail in Chapter 2).

The impacts of medical trauma and disempowering aspects of medical care are only just being recognized. Historically, compassionate communication has been left to the "bedside manner" of the healthcare provider.[27] While most healthcare providers did their utmost to provide the best care possible, some people report difficult exchanges with care providers not validating their experiences or listening to them. Sometimes this was done with the best of intentions to alleviate anxiety when the prognosis was uncertain or treatments were novel or through a lack of specialist understanding. However, having your bodily experience invalidated can be confusing, especially during childhood when your sense of self is developing. Feeling like you are not being heard is frustrating and disempowering, adding to the burden of living with a serious medical condition dependent on pioneering care. This dynamic can also indirectly communicate to us not to talk about our experiences and feelings related to our CHC, which can lead to conflicted and uncomfortable emotions. Learning to trust our bodies and communicate how we are feeling is essential to improved psychological health and well-being.

The communication skills required to deal with challenging medical situations, heightened emotions, and psychological distress are sophisticated and require specialist training. There needs to be more emphasis on this, across all healthcare professions, both embedded within training programs and as part of continual professional development. The further integration of psychologists and/or clinical social workers within medical teams would better ensure the psychological needs of the patient, family, and healthcare team are met. We will discuss this more in Chapter 12.

Thankfully, nowadays children often benefit from play therapy and access to psychological support which continues to improve for the entire family (although often still "patchy"). This was not available for many of us as pioneering children paving the way, making it even more important for us to be able to access this support and understanding in adulthood.

I remember lying in Recovery after my second heart surgery at the age of 13. I was still on a vent with so many tubes and wires coming out of my body. I was just staring at the ceiling—a ceiling covered with those soundproofing tiles with rows and rows of tiny holes. Back then our families could only visit a few minutes at a time. I was alone—just waking from major surgery, on a vent, in intense pain, and without any family with me. I just stared at the ceiling as I heard the beeping of machines in the background. As I stared at the ceiling, a young orderly came by and noticed my intense upward stare and fear. He looked at me, then he looked up at the tiles and then looked back at me. He smiled and said, "Hi, Scott. I, too, always wondered how many holes are in those tiles. Let's count the holes together." I couldn't speak, but he counted them out loud as if we were doing it together. As "we" counted the holes together, I realized that I was no longer alone—I now had a friend in the Recovery room with me. It's been 50 years, but that memory came back as if it happened yesterday. Oh yeah, in case you're wondering, there are 144 holes in each tile.

—Scott, 63 years, United States

Pioneers of the Healthcare System

At the age of 23, Julia was told by her general cardiologist that the racing heart sensation she was often experiencing was most likely just anxiety and that "many young women your age experience that sensation." She found out months later, after seeking a second opinion by a CHC specialist (and wearing a heart monitor), that she needed immediate treatment for atrial flutter, a dangerous arrhythmia.

Long-term survival of early CHC survivors was unexpected. As a result, the medical community wasn't ready to care for this growing adult population. Some of us "miracle babies" were not expected to live very long. We grew, along with medical technology, often surprising not only our families but ourselves.

Many of the early CHC survivors were either lost to follow-up care or were seen by cardiologists who did not have specialized CHC training. Today there are still not enough CHC specialists in this cardiology sub-specialty. Thanks to the Adult Congenital Heart Association in the United States, there is now an accreditation process that cardiologists and comprehensive care centers must complete in order to be deemed a specialist in this area; however, that did not occur until 2016. According to one study, even with this accreditation process, the United States is facing a likely risk of a significant shortage of ACHD board-certified physicians.[28] Meanwhile in the United Kingdom, National Health Service (which is a public health-care service) Healthcare Standards to ensure consistency of care for CHCs, driven by the Somerville Heart Foundation charity and "patient" advocacy, were introduced in England, Wales, and Northern Ireland in the early 2000s and in 2016 in Scotland.[29] While improvements are evident, globally, healthcare provision for the adult CHC population remains patchy, and there is still a lot of work to do. For example, deaths and mortality caused by congenital heart disease (CHD) were found to be the highest in low- and low–middle socioeconomic index regions of the world.[30]

As described, there is no cure for the more complex CHCs, and recent guidelines recommend lifelong monitoring.[31] Unfortunately there are fewer than 10% of adults with a CHC that are in appropriate ACHD care;[32] arguably, this is a public health crisis. When care provision has not developed in time to meet the needs of the growing population of adults with CHD, it can be inconsistent and difficult to access, especially during a medical emergency. This can add to the uncertainty of living with a CHC and leave us feeling unsafe.[33] This is why it is so important that adults are seen in a center that specializes in seeing adults with CHCs. This shortage of such specialist care provision can add to the burden of living with a complex, lifelong condition.

As a result, many adult patients continue to see pediatric cardiologists who don't usually have experience treating patients above the age of 18 years. They may end up in the waiting room with parents, children, toys, and pastel mural scenes on the walls. Others end up seeing general cardiologists who do not have the specialist training recommended to treat them. Many individual patients don't realize that not all cardiologists are the same. This difference can significantly affect a person's cardiac health and prognosis, and sometimes can be the difference between life and death. This is another reason why improving public awareness and advocacy work is so important. By working together we can improve outcomes for us all and those coming up.

Transition: Growing Out of Pediatrics

Transition from childhood to adult care providers is a time of celebration, having survived childhood with a CHC and stepping into adult life. At the same time, many individuals with a CHC have fostered a strong relationship with their pediatric cardiology team, who they may have known since birth and even credit them for saving their life. While exciting, moving on to a new care team can be unsettling and even scary, but it is vital since many pediatric cardiologists do not have training or experience in treating those over the age of 18 years.

Thankfully, transition services have improved over the last 20 years with specialized centers offering a gradual and supportive approach to transferring care between pediatric and adult services.[34] Often this was not the case for early survivors with a CHC who did not have any type of transition services to help them with the move to adult care. Many were discharged from their pediatric cardiologist and referred to a general cardiologist who was not skilled in treating CHCs.[35] In this scenario, going for follow-up appointments or being admitted to the hospital may have been associated with a new set of worries about being properly cared for and raising feelings of abandonment and loss of the only CHC cardiologist they've ever known.

Alternatively, other adults may have been discharged from pediatric care and assumed they were "cured" and no longer needed follow-up care, only to have symptoms emerge years later, propelling them into a medical crisis without a proper care team in place. One previous study revealed that one-fifth of young adults with severe CHD were not seen by a cardiologist between the ages of 18 and 22 years.[36] This lapse in care has been shown to be associated with adverse outcomes such as further cardiac complications, a greater need for urgent cardiac intervention, and an adverse impact on quality of life,[37] demonstrating the importance of this process.

Despite the undoubted progress in this area, there is still more work that needs to be done. A recent study concluded that there is still a high number of young adults who are unfortunately lost to appropriate cardiology care.[38] We will further explore this topic in Chapter 10.

Congenital Cardiology: A Growing Field

The good news is that the specialist field of congenital cardiology is growing, with more specialist centers being developed internationally, and more specialist congenital cardiologists, nurses, and other allied health professionals (such as electrophysiologists, physiotherapists, psychologists, and clinical social workers) being trained with a growing recognition of the psychological impact of living with a CHC. Certainly, we are a long way from where we need to be, but things are moving in the right direction, often as the result of combined advocacy efforts from dedicated healthcare professionals and people with lived experience. Thankfully, patient advisory committees within ACHD care centers and patient support groups are becoming more influential, while the importance of "lived experience" and "patient expertise" is increasingly being acknowledged with patient advocates working with healthcare professionals to shape care provision for future generations in many countries. As our CHC "family" grows, there are more and more outreach initiatives to help developing countries, too.

Surgical and imaging techniques, pharmacological interventions, and pain management have become more sophisticated and less invasive. Since the advance of the computer age, modern-day pacemakers and ICDs have become significantly more reliable and efficient. Additionally, biotechnology and stem cell research offer hope for even better treatments in the future.

Strong Recommendation: Specialized Care

It is now widely acknowledged that CHCs are very different from acquired heart conditions (such as coronary heart disease). As described, the American College of Cardiology and the American Heart Association,[39] the European Society of Cardiology,[40] and the NHS in the United Kingdom have designated specific care guidelines for adults with CHC which specify that there should be specialized heart centers for adult patients and that all CHC adult patients should be checked at a specialized center at least once.[41]

We were fortunate enough to speak with Paula Miller, senior education manager (and individual with a CHC) for the Adult Congenital Heart Association (ACHA) (personal interview, January 2022). Her top piece of advice for adults with CHC is to "stay in ACHD specialized care." For those living in the United States, Paula strongly recommends trying to locate an ACHA-accredited program, if possible. If not accredited, at least locate a center with cardiologists who are board certified in ACHD. She reminded us that currently only 10% of CHC patients are in specialized care. This means that 90% of those with CHCs aren't followed as per internationally recognized guidelines and are "lost to care." Paula notes there is an international shortage of ACHD specialists and that regarding her personal situation "getting into the right type of care by an ACHD specialist changed my life. I don't think I'd be here today without it." We have provided the web address for ACHA's international ACHD directory in the Appendix: Useful Organizations and Resources.

For those individuals who do not have easy access to a specialist center, sometimes they end up creating a cardiac "team," which may consist of their local, general adult cardiologist and an ACHD specialist, who they visit as recommended, sometimes less frequently, but at least once. This arrangement is usually made due to geographic location as there are fewer specialists in many rural areas. Regardless of how often you end up seeing an ACHD specialist, we recommend that they become an integral part of creating a treatment plan for your future cardiology care, and that the two physicians collaborate, as needed. This care plan will depend on a number of factors, including, but not limited to, your diagnosis, symptoms, and geographic location.

2

The Possible Impact of Having
a Congenital Heart Condition

First of all, you are not defined by your congenital heart condition (CHC). You are someone who happens to have been born with a heart condition. You matter as much as anyone else, and you are just as entitled to everything that life has to offer. We both know many individuals with a CHC that have not only survived but thrived despite their condition. The better the physical and psychological challenges of your CHC are managed, the more you will be able to embrace the other parts of yourself and your life.[1]

For some, living with a heart condition from birth can present additional challenges in life, beyond what our heart-healthy peers face. Building on the challenges discussed in Chapter 1, living with a CHC may impact many other areas of our lives, such as mental health, education, employment, finances, and relationships. We believe that in order to have the best quality of life possible, and to reach your full potential, it helps to become aware of, and open to, addressing any difficulties you may face along the way. By recognizing the challenges, you will be in a better position to make sense of the emotional and psychological impact they may have on you. This will enable you to integrate your lived experience without having to shut off parts of yourself, as can happen when we experience hardship in the absence of adequate support. This insight will put you in a better position to seek the resources you may need.

While reading this chapter, it is important to remember that not everyone faces the same difficulties; while some of the challenges described here may be relevant for you, many may not (in fact, it is highly unlikely that you will experience them all). Each of us may face these adverse experiences to a lesser or greater extent, and our resources for dealing with them will also differ greatly. Much of this depends on what else may be going on in our lives (which, of course, may change from week to week), the social and financial support available, and medical care we can access. To put it simply, everyone's situation is completely different. Even someone the same age, with the same diagnosis and medical history, could be completely different in terms of prognosis and psychosocial functioning.

Therefore, in this chapter we will be giving an overview of some of the more common challenges, and we encourage you to reflect upon and take note of anything familiar. This will hopefully help you to begin to evaluate your individual situation and, if necessary, heal and make some positive life changes. To that end, we have outlined a number of healthy coping strategies in Chapters 5–9.

Congenital Heart Conditions and Quality of Life

Before we consider the challenges, it is important to know that most people with a CHC live very full and happy lives. Much of the research shows that while there can be many psychological and emotional effects of a CHC, the majority of us thrive in terms of our ability to lead a comfortable, fulfilling, and enjoyable life, termed "quality of life." Over the past four decades, a large number of studies have been published, and the overall conclusion is that despite the increased risk of psychosocial issues, the quality of life of many adults with a CHC is actually good. People with a CHC can even have a better quality of life than their healthy peers when it is measured holistically in terms of satisfaction with life.[2]

These studies have found that the factors that impact our quality of life include the following:

- Our perception of our CHC
- Physical limitations and exercise capacity
- The quality of our social connections
- Our level of education and employment status
- Necessary treatments such as having an implantable cardiac device (e.g., implantable cardioverter-defibrillator [ICD] or pacemaker)

Another important indicator of quality of life is what is termed "sense of cohesiveness,"[3] which comprises our ability to understand, manage, accept, and derive meaning from our experiences related to our heart condition.

Further, facing lifelong adversity can make us more resilient, determined, appreciative, and able to enjoy deeper relationships, termed "post-traumatic growth,"[4] and these positive traits can also influence the quality of our lives.

Social Inequalities

When I was born with tetralogy of Fallot (TOF) in the early 1980s in Malaysia, corrective surgeries for CHDs like TOF were in its nascent stages. To save my life, my parents wrote to hospitals all over the world. So when Sir Brian Barrat-Boyes telegrammed my father to say that he would operate on me, my parents flew to New Zealand in a matter of days for my first operative interventions. Since then, CHD care in Malaysia has grown, as indicated by the establishment of the Adult Congenital Heart Disease Clinic in the National Heart Institute of Malaysia.

—Nina, 39 years old, born and raised in Malaysia

Unfortunately, children born with a CHC in low- and middle-income countries often lack access to the care they need for survival. A major barrier to progress in CHC healthcare access is the continuing "invisibility" of CHCs from the global health agenda and a lack of awareness of its prevalence and impact. CHC mortality rates decline with increasing sociodemographic index (SDI), with most deaths occurring in countries in the low- and low-to-middle SDI quintiles. Ninety percent of the world's children born with a CHC live in locations with little to no appropriate healthcare and where mortality remains high. Those with severe CHCs and without access to surgical treatment are more likely to die before their fifth birthday (although the majority who die are under the age of 1 year) compared with those in high-income countries.[5] For those who are able to access surgery, education regarding the importance of lifelong care is lacking while ongoing aftercare is often limited.[6]

Additionally, a Chilean study found that a lower household income negatively affected physical functioning and overall quality of life for people with a CHC.[7] The reason for this is uncertain; it could be that individuals living in a lower socioeconomic situation may have less opportunity for health literacy, and thus may not seek out the appropriate care and/or follow up on recommended guidelines or may face financial barriers to accessing this care (such as having to take unpaid time off work to attend appointments or recover from surgery, pay for childcare and transport to the hospital, and in countries with private healthcare having to pay for treatments and prescriptions).

In countries still struggling to fight communicable disease, children typically die undiagnosed, masking CHC's role in overall infant mortality. Due to the decrease of communicable disease, CHC has begun to emerge as a major cause of infant mortality in low- and middle-income countries.[8]

Unfortunately having a child with a congenital condition remains a stigma in many developing countries, with such children often being "hidden away" or rejected by their communities while negative attitudes about congenital conditions and cultural beliefs can present as a barrier to accessing appropriate healthcare.[9] It is important to note that such attitudinal barriers occurred, even in developed countries, until relatively recently, where for most of the 20th century children with disabilities were segregated "for their own good" in schools and institutions (if they survived).[10]

> *Being initially from an LMIC [low- and middle-income country], I believe if there was enough capacity, surgeries could be done at an earlier age, hence avoiding too many complications in adulthood. The difference is very clear as I'm currently living in a developed country where technology is topnotch, and they are able to pick up and correct complications at a very early stage.*
>
> —Magda, 33 years old, Kenya, currently living in the United States

Thankfully, there are many organizations worldwide that are involved in outreach work, partnering with local communities to perform surgeries and expand patient care through education and training, challenging stigma and advocating in the developing world. Global ARCH is an international alliance that provides outreach for people with CHCs around the world. Children's HeartLink is a US nonprofit organization that provides capacity building to pediatric heart centers.

Within the developed world, socioeconomic deprivation is linked with an increase in CHCs for a variety of reasons, while CHCs are more prevalent in black and Asian ethnic groups.[11] The factors underlying this ethnic variation are currently unclear and require further investigation. However, it is important to note the intersectionality among health, race, and social inequalities, which contribute to multiple risk factors for social exclusion and lifetime adversity.

Access to specialized care can also affect an individual's health outcome. For instance, one study reported that in the United States individuals living in rural communities are at a disadvantage in terms of their medical care due to the distance they must travel to reach a specialized care center.[12] It was also found that lower education and a lower family income can affect an individual's ability to access specialized care centers, which tend to be in urban areas.[13]

It is crucial that these social economic factors are taken into consideration when exploring CHCs and quality of life.[14]

There were no support groups when growing up and even today there are no heart rehab facilities or adult support for CHD in South Africa. A lot of what I have learnt since my fourth op in 2016 has been my own trial and error and learning, the ups and downs experiences are all self-taught."

—Andrew "Heart Warrior," 52 years old, South Africa

Barriers to Attachment

One of my most traumatic memories is of being wheeled away from my mum to the surgical theater and waking up from cardiac surgery to find she was not there because parents were not allowed in the pre-op or recovery room in the 1980s.

—Beth, 44 years old, United Kingdom

For all children, regardless of where they are born, during infancy and throughout childhood, feeling safe, loved, and cared for is essential for physical, psychological, and emotional health and development. Yet this can be more challenging for children with CHC because, for example, it is physically difficult to hold a baby who is attached to an array of medical drips and heart monitors, often in an incubator unable to breastfeed, and for some they may require a gastrostomy tube (G tube) and are unable to bottle feed. The first generation of CHC survivors' parents may not have been allowed to stay with them in the hospital or for invasive surgeries and procedures. While the importance of early attachment is now better understood, there can still, even today, be medical barriers to early bonding such as being in an incubator in a pediatric intensive care unit (PICU).

More recently, the COVID-19 pandemic made these barriers harder to overcome, with some hospital policies limiting parental access in hospitals to just one parent or even suspending this entirely. Throughout the pandemic, some hospitals prevented caregivers from accompanying their child to surgical theater or visiting them in the PICU and intensive care unit (ICU). Recent research has demonstrated a devastating impact on parent–child bonding as a result of these restrictions, with charities calling for government action to intervene and acknowledge primary caregivers as a fundamental part of a child's care team rather than a "visitor."[15]

Under normal circumstances the baby engages in a kind of biological dance with their primary caregiver (usually, but not always, their mother) using eye contact, touch, and vocalizations. When this relationship is predictable and safe, a secure bond, known as a secure attachment, develops. These early interactions shape our nervous system and provide the template on which our future relationships are built. When this relationship is healthy and consistent, over time, babies develop the capacity to regulate their own emotions and to navigate their social world. Children with a secure attachment to their primary caregivers are more resilient to traumatic life events.[16]

Yet babies with a CHC may face medical barriers to their primary caregiver, often at a time when they need them most. They may be intubated in ICUs or high-dependency wards in the hospital, attached to medical equipment. In that case it is very difficult for that biological dance to occur. When that primary attachment is interrupted in this way, it can affect an individual's ability to feel safe and secure lifelong.

It is understood that high stress or trauma experienced by infants and children early on does have an important influence on children's neural, behavioral, and psychological development, with long-lasting effects across a wide range of domains.[17] This type of adversity can be caused by an inability to access a secure, loving, consistent attachment to a primary caregiver. This may occur for a variety of medical reasons, as described, or a caregiver's inability to be present because of their own physical or mental health, which understandably may be impacted by the situation. In other words, an infant and child's early experiences, which include their relationship with their primary caregiver, can have an impact on their brain development and on how they perceive and respond to the world throughout life. For some adults with a CHC, these early experiences may still be affecting how they are coping and their overall mental health and quality of life. While early adversity can shape us in this way, healing can improve our mental health, and we can learn strategies to help us feel calmer and safer. We will explore this more in Chapter 3 and will provide coping strategies in Chapters 5–7.

Grief and Loss

Some individuals with a CHC have to deal with feelings of grief and loss very early in life. It may be because some of them had to face their own mortality at an early age. For others it may be caused by a loss of independence, certain limitations on physical abilities, or a change in health status or appearance.[18] Some women with a CHC have to face the loss of being able to safely carry a pregnancy or have a child of their own. Men can also be faced with challenging decisions about having a family due to genetic considerations and concerns about their own health. Partaking in sports, such as football, netball, or rugby is often a rite of passage for adolescents, especially among males, who often strongly identify with their team membership and develop strong, lasting friendships from such experiences. Physical restrictions that prevent people with a CHC from being able to take part, or fully engage, can result in the loss of such opportunities to make friends and to feel a sense of belonging and community that heart-healthy peers can often take for granted. Watching from the sidelines can be hard and impact negatively on self-confidence and body image, particularly for men who face cultural expectations to be strong, fit, and muscular.

It is possible to work through these feelings of grief so that we can learn to move forward and find new meaning in life. If not processed, grief can sometimes become more complicated and lead to other more serious mental health issues. We will talk in more detail about grief, loss, and healing in Chapter 4, and we have outlined different coping strategies in Chapters 5–9.

The Bigger Picture: Life Challenges

Living with a CHC can present many other challenges which reach far beyond any physical symptoms or medical interventions. These additional psychological and social challenges, known as psychosocial issues, can include feeling different; having to navigate life with a "hidden disability"; encountering problems in relationships, education, and work; and dealing with scarring and body image.[19] Living with a CHC can significantly influence adult life choices, for example about having and raising a family and which educational and career path to follow.[20]

Impact on Education, Career, and Finances

My self-esteem took quite a hit when I was little. I struggled at school and felt I was not very intelligent (not helped by a teacher calling me stupid to my face). At

school they assumed I had brain damage from being a blue baby and that it caused
my learning difficulties. Because of this no one bothered to check me for dyslexia and
giftedness, which were the actual problems. It wasn't until my second year at university
that I realised how much damage this had done to my self-esteem and that, in fact, I
wasn't "stupid" at all.

—Charlotte, 42 years old, the Netherlands

Living with a CHC can have an impact on our relationships, education, career choices, and finances, which all influence our overall quality of life. For instance, many individuals with a CHC report interruptions in education due to frequent hospitalizations. This can make it difficult for them to complete the school year or to graduate with their class of peers. In some circumstances, individuals must access special education services, hire home tutors, or attend summer school. Sometimes these interruptions prevent them from completing their college education or vocational training. People with a CHC are also at greater risk of neurocognitive difficulties, including attention-deficit/hyperactivity disorder (ADHD), which are underrecognized and underdiagnosed.[21] These experiences may single them out from their peer groups and feed into any feelings they may have about being different or not good enough. Although improving, support within the schools can unfortunately be inadequate. Increasing awareness and educating school staff is vital to promoting social inclusion and support.

For many individuals with a CHC, work is highly valued, and they are able to obtain success, despite any physical limitations. While many people with a CHC are able to work full time, it very much depends on their health status. Researchers[22] report that compared to healthy adults, even among the healthiest adults with a CHC, there are significant decrements in life expectancy, employment, and lifetime earnings. While there do seem to be limitations in employment among this population, education appears to be the main predictor for successful employment.[23] Once employed some individuals report continued interruptions and extended sick leave, as a result of ongoing CHC symptoms and treatments. While most workplaces and organizations are legally required to address workplace discrimination and promote diversity, the reality is there is often a shadow culture of health privilege.[24] Unfortunately, some people with a CHC do report experiencing workplace discrimination. In order to protect themselves, many wonder when and if they should share information about their CHC with their employers and/or coworkers. Some people report being treated poorly during a medical crisis, and having ongoing concerns about losing their job as a result. These interruptions can affect a person's entire life, reducing employability, income, health and life insurance, and their overall ability to live independently. Certainly this is not the case for everyone, and we hear many other stories about employers who are supportive and generous during medical crises.

Fortunately, most countries have employment laws to protect workers from this type of employment discrimination. For example, the US Equal Employment Opportunity Commission enforces these laws, which state that it is illegal to discriminate against someone because of their race, color, religion, sex, national origin, age, disability, or genetic information. It is important to be aware of your rights and how to access advocacy and support, and we will talk more about this in Chapter 10.

When education or employment is affected, ultimately so are a person's finances. In the United States and other countries with private healthcare systems, the availability of affordable health insurance also affects the ability to support oneself financially and make a successful transition to adulthood. Many children with a CHC have reached adulthood but in doing so can face significant challenges to achieving independence compared with their heart-healthy counterparts.[25] As a result, some individuals with a CHC report relying on their parents for transportation, financial support, medical management, and housing longer than they would have wanted, and they have a more difficult time launching into the next phase of adulthood. Studies have found that parental attitudes and parental overprotectiveness can also influence their child's ability to launch.[26] Alternatively, some have reported needing to accept jobs they otherwise would not have in order to secure the company's health insurance coverage.

Hidden Scars: Feeling Different and Discrimination

Jennifer's colleagues got into running. They would all go for a run during their lunch hour or after work and sign up for different races together. They would talk about it endlessly, comparing distances, personal best times, and injuries with each other. They all knew about her CHC but presumably because she looked young and fit it never crossed their minds how left out she felt, and how far their reality was from hers.

Many of us grew up feeling really lucky. We benefited from brand-new medical technology which enabled us to survive. While this is pretty significant, we cannot forget that it can come at a cost. Some individuals have had to undergo invasive, painful, repeated interventions and hospitalizations dating back to childhood. These experiences can be traumatic and, for some, they can affect the way they see themselves and the world around them. As children, some of them may also have witnessed the suffering of others on their hospital ward, during hospital appointments and medical tests.

Since most individuals with a CHC are diagnosed at birth, having a serious, chronic illness is their normal, and they know nothing else. Further, many have never had the opportunity to meet another individual with a CHC and that made it more likely for them to feel different from their peers or not good enough. This may have led to them hiding their condition or overcompensating to "fit in."

Those who did have the opportunity to meet other people with a CHC often report positive experiences in meeting someone "like me." Depending on the situation, sometimes those meetings can be troubling if the other individual has a different health status or prognosis. It can be scary if that other individual is not doing as well as you are health-wise. One may leave that meeting worried: "Will that (deteriorating health) happen to me?" or possibly feeling a sense of survivor's guilt: "Why am I doing better physically than they are when we have the same diagnosis?" Alternatively, if they are doing better than you physically, you might feel upset that things haven't worked out so well for you. If you do have the opportunity to meet another individual with a similar CHC, we suggest going into that meeting with the knowledge that even with a similar health history, everyone is different, and comparison is usually not helpful.

> *After attending genetic counseling, Amy and her husband, Duncan, decided not to have a family. They felt the risks were too high for Amy and the baby. It wasn't an easy decision, but they both felt it was right for them. Years later Amy met someone with the same heart condition as her through a patient support group. When they told her they had two children, she felt upset and angry, and she started to question her decision. She reached out for support from a therapist, who helped her to work through her grief.*

While today most cases of CHC are diagnosed in utero or at birth, there are some individuals who are diagnosed with their CHC later in childhood or even adulthood. Some may have been diagnosed during a routine medical exam. Others may have experienced cardiac symptoms prompting evaluation or had a heart-related event which required emergency medical attention. This understandably can be shocking and very difficult, especially if surgical intervention is recommended. Sometimes a diagnosis is made, and there is no need for any intervention. Other times follow-up, medication, further testing, or surgery is recommended. Depending on the situation, there could be some trauma involved, as in the case of an unexpected cardiac event. In this case, individuals will need time to process and share their wide array of feelings about all that has happened in a safe environment. It is normal to feel a loss of health status and to go through a period of adjustment to and acceptance of their newly diagnosed CHC. Much of what we talk about in this book in regards to mood and coping is relevant in this situation.

My heart journey is quite different from most of my peers in the heart world. Unlike the majority of them, I did not grow up knowing I had a congenital heart defect. I was completely blindsided by the diagnosis, which immediately sent me into a tailspin of depression. I wasn't even 30 years old, and I was facing open heart surgery. In the 3 months between diagnosis and surgery, I tried just about every method out there to get through the mental darkness that I was experiencing. I've learned that I'll never be able to delete those memories from 5 years ago, but I can use that traumatic situation to help others. Now that I'm recovered, I've been able to connect with numerous individuals facing either the same diagnosis or heart surgery in general. I've been able to offer a level of comfort that I only wish I'd been able to find when I was diagnosed.
                                                                    —Katherine, 35 years old, United States

People with a CHC often describe growing up feeling different from their peers,[27] which sometimes stems from their childhood. We may have explicitly been told that we are different, labeled a "miracle baby" or "special" by adults around us, and we may at times have been treated as a "medical curiosity." From an early age we may have sensed anxiety from our parents and adults taking care of us and a feeling that something is "wrong" with us because we were treated differently than our peers.

Further, our experience of childhood may have been different from our heart-healthy peers. Some individuals describe missing a lot of school, physical activities, or socializing with peers due to their CHC. For some, gaps in education caused them to repeat grades, further isolating them from their peers, or sadly they may never have been addressed due to the uncertainty of their long-term survival. Some describe feeling embarrassed by not being chosen for sports teams, not being allowed to participate in physical education class, or being unable to take part in active play. For others, this underlying feeling of not being "normal" (Is there really such a thing?) or not being good enough may stem from surgical scarring, physical differences such as being smaller in stature, internal cardiac devices, or cyanosis. Some individuals describe being left out, teased, or bullied as a result of these physical differences, for example by not being invited to parties or trips because other parents were frightened about feeling responsible for us, being teased for having "blue lips," or having to wear a 24-hour heart monitor in class.

All of these experiences have the risk of greatly affecting an individual's body image, self-esteem, and overall self-confidence. For children it is important to feel a part of their peer group, and feeling left out can be difficult and confusing. It is also completely normal for children to compare themselves with their friends and other children. As teenagers begin to develop their emerging, independent identities, they are especially sensitive to not fitting in and appearing different. To fit in, some individuals try to conceal their heart condition. Some have even gone as far as using makeup on a new surgical scar, at the risk of causing dangerous infection. Others report concealing their CHC so they aren't treated differently, "babied," labeled ("the girl with the heart condition"), or treated with kid gloves. However, this can lead to other difficulties, such as having to mask symptoms (potentially damaging our health), hiding scars, and ultimately feeling like an imposter.

Conversely, some individuals report feeling frustrated because their CHC is "hidden," which makes it harder for other heart-healthy individuals to understand or at times even believe their physical limitations. This can put them in the uncomfortable situation of having to frequently explain why they are unable to go with the flow and do everything their heart-healthy peers do. Some examples include not being able to walk safely through certain metal detectors (if they have an implanted device) or participate in certain sports. Or why they might need to take frequent rests, take medication multiple times per day, or have a disability parking sticker. We have heard of individuals being reprimanded by random strangers (and sometimes acquaintances) for displaying a disability parking sticker on their car and using it when they "look perfectly young and healthy."

Learning to communicate with others about your condition and your needs is important as is your relationship with yourself, and we will discuss this more in Chapter 8. We will also consider issues around self-managing a "hidden" health condition in Chapter 10.

Hospital Visits, Medical Procedures, and Cardiac Events

Visiting my cardiologist as an adult is really stressful. I'm always scared that this is going to be the appointment where they tell me I'm in active heart failure or something. To cope, I always take the entire day off from work in case they order extra tests (which they often do), or in case I just need to go home and be by myself afterwards. I usually end up listening to an audiobook or working on a puzzle while waiting to be seen. This helps me to unwind.

—Lenea, 33 years old, United States

Sometimes something as "simple" as visiting your cardiologist for a regular follow-up appointment can raise mixed emotions. The visit may bring up memories from past medical experiences and/or remind us of our fears about the future. It is important to know this is common; however, these appointments are also your opportunity to manage your healthcare, ask questions, and develop a positive working relationship with your medical team. It is important that as adults, we are the captain of our ship, or, in other words, that we take charge of the direction of our healthcare. Many individuals report that choosing and partnering with your adult congenital heart disease (ACHD) team really does help in getting through not only your medical appointments but also any stressful health-related situations that may arise. For many adults with a CHC, it is necessary to return to the hospital for follow-up interventions or surgeries.

Having to return to where you have previously experienced difficult news, painful interventions, and felt unwell can be particularly challenging. Often we are asked to strip off our clothing for medical examinations or procedures. We might be asked to wear a revealing backless hospital gown, which can leave us feeling even more vulnerable, exposed, cold, and feeling in the "patient role."[28] It can make things particularly hard when we know that we will likely have to endure these procedures again, as in the case of those with implantable devices.

We can also have mixed feelings about these visits, too. We may have spent a lot of time in the hospital as children, which may almost feel like a "second home." We may have built up strong relationships with our care team and look forward to seeing them. We may also have happy memories of times with people who have tried their best to take care of us when we needed it most and made us feel better. We may feel "safer" and in the best hands in the hospital when we are unwell or grateful for the rest if we have been battling through everyday life having to manage fatigue or other debilitating symptoms. We may feel relieved and hopeful that something is going to be done to make us feel better and enable us to reclaim our lives, such as a cardiac device change, ablation, or transplant. Some individuals have even reported that after long hospital stays, it was hard to go home to face "the real world" and life's other stressors after living in the "safety bubble" of the hospital micro-community with their care team on hand.

At the same time, medical procedures are often experienced as painful and frightening. They can be overwhelming, cause feelings of helplessness, and may give a sense of life threat.[29] Some of the reasons a CHC patient may need to be hospitalized include cardiac surgery, need for a pacemaker or implantable cardiac defibrillator (ICD) cardiac ablation, arrhythmia, or medication adjustment. Sometimes hospitalization occurs suddenly, as in the cases of certain arrhythmias, stroke, and cardiac arrest. All of these reasons can understandably contribute to feelings of anxiety and trigger symptoms of posttraumatic stress.[30] It can be frightening to experience these cardiac symptoms, especially when they may indicate a worsening of our condition or that further medical explorations or interventions may be required. Heart symptoms might trigger feelings of anxiety (and vice versa) if similar feelings in the past have indicated a serious problem (see Chapters 5 and 9 for more on this).

> *Be it our hot, humid wedding day, helping friends move into a new house or simply lifting my young children, my activities were significantly limited by the risk that they would trigger tachycardia or atrial flutter, ultimately requiring a cardioversion to restore normal rhythm. This weighed heavily on me and even following a successful ablation, and now 20 years later, that dark cloud is still included in every equation.*
>
> —Mitch, 59 years old, United States

Dealing with "cardiac events" or other symptoms at any age can be challenging for people with a CHC. These can include heart palpitations such as irregular beats, feeling as if your heart is beating too fast or slow or feeling dizzy or light-headed. This can be particularly scary and sometimes confusing as it isn't always easy to know if these changes in rhythm warrant a call to your cardiologist or a hospital visit. It can be difficult to know which cardiac events merit further medical exploration and which to ignore. It is important to discuss these concerns with your medical team to get advice about how to tell the difference and have a plan of action should you need to make a call.

Some individuals with a CHC require implantable cardiac devices. Learning to live with an implantable device can be challenging, both physically as well as psychologically. For those with a mechanical valve, the clicking sound can sometimes create complicated feelings. For some, it is distracting and sometimes upsetting, and for others, in time it is something they grow used to and don't even notice or find reassuring. Individuals with implantable pacemakers or implantable cardioverter-defibrillators (ICDs) live with the knowledge that the battery, and less frequently the leads, of these devices must be changed, which requires additional surgeries throughout their lives. Additionally, for those with ICDs they often have concerns about being shocked by the device going off, which can also create worry for some people. Living with a cardiac device for people with a CHC can be more complicated because they likely have depended on one from a much younger age than people with acquired heart conditions.[31] For example, they may face issues with lead extraction, occlusion (blocking) of veins with multiple leads, scarring, and finding space for multiple devices across the lifespan. This can lead to misconceptions about "only having a pacemaker" from medical staff, complex pacing issues, and issues accessing the specialist care required. Other physical concerns that can add to the burden of living with a CHC can include side effects from certain medications, regular International Normalized Ratio (INR) testing for those taking anticoagulation medications, and managing swollen ankles and fluid retention. For some individuals with a CHC, their only treatment option is to have a heart transplant. Some have gone through the stressful evaluation process, and others live with the knowledge that transplant may be in their not-so-distant future.

It is normal to have a wide variety of feelings when dealing with new symptoms, hospitalizations, or finding out you need to have surgery. These feelings may include, but not be limited to, sadness, fear, anger, frustration, or anxiety. The good news is that when dealing with these medical situations, there are many things we can do to help ourselves through these stressful events (in Chapter 5–9) and to get the support that we need.

COVID-19: "The Great Equalizer"

The year 2020 brought a new challenge for those of us living with a CHC: the global COVID-19 pandemic. Despite talk of the pandemic being a "great equalizer," in reality it has intensified health inequalities, with the most vulnerable facing the greatest impact physically, psychologically, economically, and socially.[32] The pandemic has also had a profound impact on health and social care workers who provide our care,[33] increasing levels of stress, moral injury, and burnout for them.

The pandemic also presents increased risk to mental health for people with underlying health conditions. Studies have reported disruption to cardiac care during the pandemic for the CHC population, concerns about infection, and high levels of psychological distress in the CHC population, across the lifespan.[34] Yet one study also found that while people with a CHC report elevated levels of posttraumatic stress disorder (PTSD) on a screening measure during the pandemic, many also report being able to draw from their lifelong experience of living with medical uncertainty to cope.[35] In many ways the CHC population has been well placed to manage this global health crisis.

Living with Uncertainty about Prognosis

There are real challenges in ACHD clinical practice given the lack of published evidence compared to the other areas in cardiology.

—ACHD cardiologist, United Kingdom

Living with a CHC often means living with uncertainty. Individuals will often hear their cardiologist say, "We aren't sure," or "We've never had a patient at your age with your condition." As human beings, it is perfectly normal to have different emotions when hearing this, which may include stress, anxiety, and sadness. It is vital that we are able to recognize these feelings and connect them to their trigger so that we can better process and manage them.

The Perfect Storm: Mental Health

Recently I have been fighting breast cancer and at every turn you get offered psychological help. In all my 42 years I have never been offered that in relation to my heart disease.

—Charlotte, 42 years old, The Netherlands

We've talked about the unique challenges that living with a CHC can bring and how this can create the "perfect storm," putting us at higher risk of developing symptoms of depression, anxiety, or posttraumatic stress. We know from studies that 50% of individuals with a CHC met diagnostic criteria for a lifetime mood or anxiety disorder,[36] which is more than double the prevalence found in the general public.[37] Another study found that 79% of adults with a CHC had a diagnosable psychiatric illness, yet none of those individuals were receiving any mental health treatment.[38]

Yet, unfortunately, it seems that many individuals with a CHC "suffer silently and worry alone."[39] One study reported that approximately 69% of the patients who met diagnostic criteria for a mood or anxiety disorder at the time of their interview were not engaged in any type of mental health treatment,[40] while another revealed that it was common for mental health disorders in the CHC adult population to be missed or undiagnosed.[41]

Yet the development of mental health difficulties as a result of living with a CHC is not inevitable. There are many ways in which these outcomes could be prevented, mitigated, and treated. Why is this so important? Not only is it distressing and painful to live with psychological or emotional issues, it also can have a negative impact on functioning. Research has demonstrated a connection between mental and physical health. Specifically, studies on individuals with acquired heart disease found that those with depression have worse physical outcomes, resulting in more deaths and repeated cardiovascular events.[42] Other studies report PTSD is a risk factor for heart disease,[43] and individuals with depression or PTSD were found to have a higher likelihood of noncompliance with their physician's recommendations.[44]

The good news is that there are effective, evidence-based treatments for mental health difficulties, including psychological therapies and psychotropic medications, while evidence suggests that treating them may actually help the heart.[45] We also know more than ever before about the impact of adverse and traumatic life events on the brain and body, how to employ protective factors to mitigate their impact, and coping strategies to help us to manage difficult feelings, thoughts, and behaviors. We want you to benefit from this knowledge to help to address the psychological impact.

Perfect Storm Case Study: Donald

Donald is a 30-year-old teacher from England. He was born with a heart condition requiring open heart surgery as an infant, and again when he was 8 years old. Generally speaking, he feels well and he doesn't think much about his condition, although he is aware that he may need further surgery and possibly a pacemaker one day. He doesn't really speak about his health, and when anyone else does, he brushes it off with a joke. He has some hazy memories of being in the ICU as a child, but for the most part remembers the hospital as somewhere he has always gone for an annual checkup and some mildly inconvenient tests.

When he enters his early 30s, he experiences frequent arrhythmia, which, as a result, requires several emergency room visits for cardioversions and medication trials, occurring over a 3-year span. During one of his emergency room visits, it becomes necessary for him to have surgery to fit a pacemaker right away, with little time to process it emotionally.

After his discharge, Donald starts to feel panicky about his heart health and starts to monitor his heart rate regularly throughout the day. He begins to have distressing dreams and flashbacks about being a young child in the hospital. One day he has a panic attack during which he struggles to breathe, feels hot and sweaty, and thinks he is going to collapse. He is convinced that he is having a heart attack. Despite being given the "all clear" at the hospital, he stops socializing or exerting himself and dreads going out in case it happens again. He feels annoyed with himself and berates himself for "not coping" when he has always been so "strong." He delays his return to work yet worries about finances and whether he will ever be able to work again. He struggles to share his worries with his friends and family, and some of them notice a change in his usual outgoing personality. At the suggestion of his girlfriend, Donald reluctantly begins therapy for the first time.

Through therapy Donald's fears are heard and validated. This offers him a chance to share his real feelings and concerns without having to worry about upsetting anyone that he is close to. He is encouraged to meet with his CHC team to address his concerns, including future pacemaker surgeries, symptoms to look out for, how to access specialist care in an emergency, what he can expect in terms of future family planning, and whether it is safe to have sex. This meeting helps him to feel more empowered and in control. He begins to feel a sense of relief by sharing his emotions with someone supportive and objective. In therapy he learns grounding exercises, breathing techniques, and guided imagery, and many of his negative thoughts are gently challenged and replaced by a more realistic and positive perspective. Donald learns about how anxiety affects the mind and body and creates coping statements, or mantras, to help him manage it. He works with his therapist to process some of the medical trauma he experienced and starts to trust his body again. In turn, he gradually starts to socialize more, which helps to rebuild his confidence and improve his mood. He is able to resume intimacy with his girlfriend after sharing his concerns with her about his scar and reassurance from his medical team about physical activity.

At the suggestion of his therapist he reaches out to a congenital heart organiza-
tion where he meets some new friends with CHCs. This helps to normalize his
experience, and he begins to feel less alone. The organization is also able to offer him
advice about financial assistance and employment rights. In turn, he begins to talk
more openly about his condition to wider family, friends, and colleagues and to share
the unique challenges he faces. This helps him "fill in the gaps" about some of his
early experiences, make sense of his triggers, and become more accepting of his health
situation.

Donald and his therapist mutually agree that he no longer needs the extra sup-
port of therapy. He continues to work on himself by improving his self-care, which
helps him to build his confidence. He also becomes more self-compassionate instead
of comparing himself to his heart-healthy peers and berating himself when he feels
"different." Instead of feeling ashamed when he can't "keep up," he understands
that he faces challenges his peers don't and he feels proud of how he manages them.
He recognizes that his tendency to withdraw when he is upset makes him feel more
isolated, and he begins to reach out more for support rather than letting things bottle
up. He starts to recognize how his health condition helps him prioritize what really
matters to him, and he increases his appreciation for his life and loved ones. When
he feels ready, he speaks with his employers and arranges a phased return to work.
While he recognizes there may be challenges ahead, he feels positive about his future
and better equipped and supported to deal with what comes his way.

Emotional distress is a normal reaction to tough life events. Yet there is
not always the opportunity to process these feelings when dealing with
this serious lifelong medical condition. Of course, not everyone who has
grown up with a heart condition will experience these feelings or issues.
We are all unique, with different personalities, diagnosis, medical interventions, complications, prognoses, and life circumstances. Despite these
challenges, there are strategies which may help you to cope in a healthy
way. Of course, you bring your own wisdom, having dealt with your condition, possibly for many years. Here, we hope to build on this, to help
you process what you may not have had the time or the opportunity to
deal with and to create a space to demystify and manage the very real
emotional and psychological response to living with a serious lifelong
health condition.

As psychotherapists who have benefited from pioneering congenital cardiac care, our life experiences and education have helped us to live well

with a lifelong heart condition. We hope to empower and to equip you with insight, guidance, and healthy coping strategies. We also want you to know that you are not alone in your experience as an adult living with a congenital heart condition. First, let's explore further how anxiety and trauma can affect our mind and body.

3

Understanding the Body's Alarm System

Anxiety and Trauma

Everyone feels anxious at times. Anxiety is a normal response to uncertainty and to situations that we find threatening or challenging. Sometimes anxiety can be useful if it motivates us to make positive changes and take action toward solving a problem, such as studying for a big exam or gathering the courage to make a positive life change. However, it can become a problem when we feel anxious a lot of the time and when it begins to negatively affect our lives.

Research has consistently shown that as individuals with congenital heart conditions (CHCs), we have a higher likelihood of developing an anxiety disorder.[1] This is understandable, given all that we have to endure medically and beyond. It can be overwhelming dealing with a serious medical condition while trying to respond to everyday "normal" stressors (e.g., bills, work, or family issues). Yet stress and anxiety are seldom screened for by medical professionals, and they often have limited resources to treat them. As a result, issues with anxiety often go undetected, which is unfortunate because there are many treatment options. Learning how to manage anxiety can greatly improve our overall quality of life and physical health. In this chapter we will explain what anxiety is, its connection to having a CHC, and how for some it can develop into an anxiety disorder.

Living with a CHC often means that we have to cope with a lot of uncertainty. Many of the situations we are faced with are unexpected and are outside of the usual range of human experience. We have summarized some examples of these situations in Figure 3.1. This list is not exhaustive; there may be some situations that you have encountered that we have not

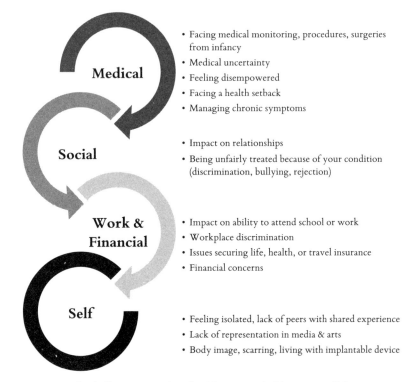

Medical
- Facing medical monitoring, procedures, surgeries from infancy
- Medical uncertainty
- Feeling disempowered
- Facing a health setback
- Managing chronic symptoms

Social
- Impact on relationships
- Being unfairly treated because of your condition (discrimination, bullying, rejection)

Work & Financial
- Impact on ability to attend school or work
- Workplace discrimination
- Issues securing life, health, or travel insurance
- Financial concerns

Self
- Feeling isolated, lack of peers with shared experience
- Lack of representation in media & arts
- Body image, scarring, living with implantable device

Figure 3.1 Life challenges associated with congenital heart conditions.

included, and we encourage you to acknowledge any that we may have missed. Reading this list may bring up difficult memories or make you feel anxious or overwhelmed. If it does trigger anxiety or other uncomfortable feelings, then we encourage you to express them either through journaling, talking to someone you trust, or drawing from the tools and techniques described in Chapters 5–9.

As the situations listed are often unique to individuals with a CHC, one factor which can make them even more challenging is that our day-to-day peer group is not going through the same experiences. This provides very little opportunity to share and make sense of how you are feeling. It is part of our human nature to process and attempt to understand what has happened to us by sharing our experiences with our family and friends. When we don't have this opportunity, we can feel isolated and may even begin to feel different. You may also feel that it is unfair that you have to endure these experiences when your social group does not. This might make you feel understandably anxious, resentful, and angry at times. If this is the case, it can be helpful to meet other individuals with a CHC.[2]

If you decide to reach out to a CHC peer, please remember that everyone's CHC experience is different. You may connect to someone who is of similar age, with the same diagnosis, but your two experiences may be completely different. Just because one person has faced a specific challenge, it does not mean everyone will. This awareness is crucial to having a positive peer connection experience. We have listed support organizations in the Appendix that can help link you with CHC peers.

It is hardly surprising that when faced with these stressful situations, in the context of limited support, our body's alarm system may be triggered. When this alarm system is activated, feelings of anxiety begin. It is helpful to have a good understanding of what your personal alarm system is, how it feels in your body so that you can recognize when it has been activated, and to develop techniques that you can use to manage it and turn it back off.

The Body's Alarm System: Fight, Flight, or Freeze Response

As mammals, we have evolved to respond quickly to protect ourselves from predators and other dangers. Many of the symptoms of anxiety are part of our body's alarm system, which is triggered when we feel under threat.[3] When the alarm system in our body switches on, we are going into defense mode.

This alarm response is driven by our autonomic nervous system, which includes nerves that carry messages between our brain and body. When there is a perceived threat, an arm of that system, called the sympathetic nervous system, takes over. This is the system in our body which prepares us to respond quickly in order to keep ourselves safe. When this is activated, it redirects blood flow to our major organs and muscle groups (to better enable us to "escape" from the threat), and it also increases our breathing and our heart rates. Simply stated, when we go into fight or flight mode, our body is preparing for action by taking in more oxygen. In this event, the big muscles in our body get ready to fight or flee the situation. In the modern world, we don't usually have to physically fight or flee predators, and we may instead be left with our bodies feeling charged and tense. Over time this can lead to back, neck, and head pain and tension. Since blood is directed away from our digestive system, we may also feel nauseous or experience digestive discomfort.

When the blood flow is redirected (remember the blood flow was redirected to the larger muscles and organs), we often don't have the ability to think the situation through. In this state individuals may report brain "fog," an inability to focus, and they may find it harder to think clearly. Some people report not being able to think of anything except the anxiety, fear, or terror.

This increase in heart rate and breathing occasionally can develop into rapid "over breathing" known as hyperventilation. When someone hyperventilates, they often report feeling dizzy or breathless and describe that their heart is racing. This can occur when our bodies detect a danger, even when it isn't really there, and sometimes it can develop into what is called a panic attack. During a panic attack, individuals often report having thoughts like *I am having a heart attack, I am going to collapse, I am going to make a fool of myself,* or *Am I dying?* What they don't realize is that the alarm system is stuck in the "on" position, which is causing their symptoms; it is a healthy bodily response, just at the wrong time. We will explore a range of tools through Chapters 5–7 that can help unstick it.

These physiological changes in response to perception of threat or danger explain why when you are feeling anxious you may notice many changes in how your body feels. Although the fight or flight mode is actually a healthy response to threat, often people do not understand what is happening to their body (which will then affect their mind). This lack of understanding can make them feel even more anxious, leading to a vicious cycle of anxiety, worrying thoughts, and physical symptoms. In turn, often they may turn to quick-fix safety behaviors (such as rushing back home, avoiding certain places or situations, or seeking reassurance) that can actually keep the problem going in the longer term.

As grown adults, almost everyone must deal with traffic, paying bills, office politics, and so on, but in these situations it is unnecessary (and unhelpful) for us to go into fight or flight mode. However, as individuals with a CHC, we still do face occasional real threats, such as medical procedures, awaiting medical test results, or responding to other unexpected cardiac symptoms. In these cases we don't need to run away from danger; in fact, usually what we need is a clear and focused mind to make decisions and stay calm which will help us to get through the challenge we are facing.

Feelings	**Thoughts**	**Physical Symptoms**	**Behavior**
Anxiety	Racing	Nausea	Urge to act
Panic	Catastrophizing	Shaky	Urge to escape
Dread	Brain fog	Heart racing	(evade danger)
Anger	Decreased memory	Breathlessness	Urge to fight
	"Something terrible will	Muscle tension	
	happen"	Sweaty	
	"I might collapse/die"	Agitated	
	"I'll make a fool of myself"		
	"I have no control"		

Figure 3.2 Fight, flight, or freeze: how the mind and body respond to threat.

When our nervous system is stuck in this heightened response mode, it elevates levels of stress hormones called cortisol and adrenaline in our body. Chronic elevated levels of cortisol have been linked to increases in weight gain and decreased immune function, and they can have detrimental effects on your overall health, both physically and psychologically.[4] Prolonged elevated cortisol levels may impact sleep, cognitive function (our ability to think clearly and our memory), appetite, and mood. This is why it is so important to know the triggers which ignite your alarm system and learn healthy coping strategies to help you stay within your window of tolerance. Figure 3.2 depicts common symptoms of fight or flight.

Sometimes I Just Freeze: Hypoarousal Response

Sometimes, if we feel like our life is at risk, rather than feeling compelled to act we become immobilized, feel numb, and may dissociate (feel detached from our body). This is known as hypoarousal. In contrast to the fight or flight response described earlier, during this "freeze" response our body "shuts down" rather than being activated. This is because the body is "playing dead" for survival rather than preparing to fight or flee the danger because this seems like the best option at the time. Afterward, we may struggle to recall what happened to us because the parts of our brain that make sense of events and store memories are shut down. For example, this may happen during invasive hospital procedures where you have no control, are unable to move, and feel very scared and vulnerable. If this happens to you, then grounding exercises and breathing techniques can help to bring you back to the present moment, while taking yourself to a safe space in your mind can help to return your body to a place of calm. We will cover these strategies in Chapters 5–7.

Threat Response: Window of Tolerance

Trauma disorders reflect a nervous system that is biased to cues of danger rather than safety, reflecting a perilous history.

—Ogden and Fisher (2018)[5]

One way to think about how the body responds to a threat is depicted in Figure 3.3. To feel healthy, we need to be able to assess and respond to our

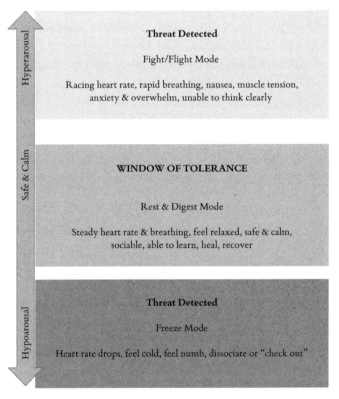

Figure 3.3 Window of tolerance (adapted from Porges 2018)[6].

How the body responds to a threat. Repeated exposure to traumatic situations during development can lead to a smaller window of tolerance for feeling calm and increased reactivity to stressors.

environment when we are both safe and unsafe. The goal is to stay within the window of tolerance, which is when we feel calm, relaxed, and safe most of the time.[7]

If we experience a lot of trauma when we are growing up, we may be more likely to interpret situations as threatening. This makes sense: if you are raised in a more "hostile" environment, it is important for your survival to have a more responsive threat system for protection. In that case, our window of tolerance when we feel safe and secure becomes smaller and more reactive to stressors. This may be the case for some of us with CHCs since we may face exposure to potentially traumatic early life events, such as surgery, poor health, and medical barriers to bonding with our caregivers. These factors can affect how we react to and manage stress. In turn, as social animals, this can influence our relationships, as we need to feel safe most of the time for healthy social connection to take place. It is possible to widen your window of tolerance over time by practicing grounding, relaxation, and mindfulness techniques and somatic exercises, which we will explore in Chapters 5–7.

Heart–Mind Link

Since the heart is central to our nervous system, any heart problems may affect how efficiently our bodies respond to threats. This could, in part, explain why people with a CHC are at greater risk of anxiety and posttraumatic stress disorder (PTSD).[8] Further, studies have identified emotional stress and poor psychological health[9] with increased risk of cardiovascular events. This heart–mind connection is important to be aware of as it will hopefully motivate us to address our uncomfortable emotions and overall mental health.

To this end, dealing with anxiety is critical as it can affect how we think, how we feel, and how we behave. If not properly addressed, in some cases it can potentially develop into a more extreme form of anxiety such as panic disorder, health anxiety, phobias, or PTSD. Next we describe some of the more common ways anxiety is expressed when dealing with a CHC, but it is in no way exhaustive of all of the ways some people experience it.

It is also important to know that there are some underlying physical conditions which can contribute to symptoms of anxiety. If you are experiencing a lot of anxiety, it is recommended that you have a thorough medical evaluation to rule out the possibility of a physical cause. For instance, certain medications, an overactive thyroid, and hormones are just some of the possible contributing factors. If there is an underlying cause and it is not identified and treated, then the anxiety will most likely continue or get worse. Another potential contributor to anxiety is a genetic predisposition. Having a family member with anxiety doesn't automatically mean you will develop it; however, it is important to give a thorough family history to your healthcare provider if you seek treatment.

Health Anxiety and Heart-Focused Anxiety

I had a lot of anxiety after getting my pacemaker. During that time, I could not fall asleep unless I was taking my pulse. I was afraid that my pacemaker would stop working. I was so afraid my heart would stop, too. I wasn't able to sleep without performing this ritual. I knew it wasn't healthy, but I couldn't help it.

—Alex, 54 years old, United States

Anxiety is a very physical emotion that specifically affects the heart, causing our heart rate to either speed up (during fight or flight) or slow down (during freeze), and which can also cause palpitations and even chest pain. For people living with a CHC, all of these sensations can mimic symptoms that previously indicated cardiac problems such as arrhythmia, a fault with your pacemaker or implantable cardioverter-defibrillator (ICD), or an overall worry that something else is wrong with your heart, making it difficult to tell the difference between anxiety-induced heart flutters and more serious issues.

This can lead to a vicious cycle where you become hypervigilant about cardiac symptoms. This can develop into "safety-seeking" behaviors such as constantly scanning your body for symptoms, having an inability to fully focus on anything else, and avoiding things that may trigger symptoms or uncomfortable feelings (such as physical exertion). During this time, you may also seek reassurance from family, friends, or healthcare providers. However, if you come to rely too much on this, it can feed the anxiety, undermine your confidence, and impact your life and day-to-day functioning. The confusing part for the individual with a CHC is that sometimes the symptoms are related to a health crisis. The only way to be certain is to seek a medical evaluation to rule out a physical problem.

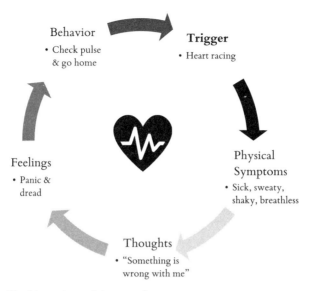

Figure 3.4 Health anxiety vicious cycle.

Once a physical cause is ruled out, then the challenge is learning to use tools (such as grounding, breathing exercises, coping statements) to decrease the anxiety, lower the adrenaline, and steady the breath so that the symptoms subside while gradually challenging avoidance and reassurance seeking and building up your confidence in your body (as described in Chapters 5–7).

If this health-related worry or anxiety gets out of control, it can lead to a condition called health anxiety. When the focus is on anxiety and the heart, this is known as heart-focused health anxiety,[10] which is experienced by some CHC patients (see Figure 3.4).

Panic Disorder

Anxiety can sometimes manifest in a group of symptoms called a panic attack. This occurs when the body's alarm system is triggered due to a false threat. Basically, the alarm system goes off when we do not need, want, or expect it to, often triggered by a traumatic reminder or an accumulation of stressors. During a panic attack,[11] individuals may experience symptoms such as a racing heart rate, chest pain, rapid breathing, sweating, nausea, and brain fog. While these symptoms are actually a normal part of the fight, flight, or freeze response, people often report that during a panic attack they believe they are at risk of dying, collapsing, or making a fool of themselves. Panic attacks are debilitating, and after experiencing one many individuals worry about it happening again and start to avoid anything they associate as a trigger (such as the place where it happened or what they were doing at the time). However, this can get in the way of daily life and develop into a vicious cycle. If this is an issue for you, it is important that you first see a doctor to rule out an underlying physical reason for your symptoms. Once ruled out, it is important to know that during a panic attack you are experiencing a healthy, normal response to perceived threat, just at the wrong time. There are things you can do to treat this type of anxiety, to turn your nervous system to the off position (see Chapters 5– 7), reduce background stressors, challenge avoidance behaviors, and quell catastrophic thoughts.

Posttraumatic Stress Disorder

> *Trauma is not what happens to us but what we hold inside in the absence of an empathic witness.*
>
> —Peter Levine, *Waking the Tiger*[12]

Those of us with CHCs may experience adverse and traumatic life events such as invasive, repeated, and unexpected medical procedures, surgeries, and difficult health news sometimes in the absence of loved ones. It is essential to note that experiencing a traumatic event does not mean that you will develop a trauma disorder. In fact, most people who experience a traumatic event do not.

Following exposure to a traumatic incident, it is quite common to replay the event in your mind, often as nightmares and flashbacks. This is how our minds make sense of what has happened to us, especially if we were too overwhelmed to process what was going on at the time. Following these challenging situations, it is also common and understandable to feel anxious, angry, guilty, and sad. We may experience difficulty sleeping and continue to feel on guard after the situation is over. Often we try to avoid reminders of the trauma to block out thinking about it.

All of these signs are a normal response to an unusually difficult situation. Usually, they will fade in the days and weeks after the event. Sometimes they persist and develop into a more serious anxiety disorder known as posttraumatic stress disorder (PTSD).[13] Often this happens because we did not have the resources we needed during and after the traumatic event to process what was happening to us. Many of the symptoms of PTSD are a normal response to trauma that don't "switch off." If they persist or get worse for more than 1 month after the traumatic incident, however, it is recommended that you seek treatment.

The recognition of "trauma disorders" originates from studies of soldiers' response to combat during World War I. Originally termed "shell shock," it became evident that some soldiers who had been exposed to prolonged and intense attacks developed psychological symptoms. At the time this was poorly managed and understood with many being stigmatized and labeled deserters. Understanding has thankfully improved, and PTSD is now a recognized medical condition. Further, it is now accepted that PTSD is not exclusive to veterans and can occur in response to other traumatic life events in civilian populations.

PTSD can include symptoms such as hypervigilance, difficulty sleeping, poor concentration, low mood, decreased interest in things you previously enjoyed, self-blame, emotional and physical reactivity after exposure to traumatic reminders (often sensory in nature, such as smells and sounds), and reliving of the traumatic event as nightmares and/or flashbacks. Flashbacks are when we respond to past events as if they are happening in the here and now, rather than unpleasant memories from the past.

Complex PTSD can develop following repeated, interpersonal, and often childhood traumatic events. Symptoms include pervasive shame and guilt, difficulty regulating emotions, dissociation, relationship difficulties, and engaging in risky behaviors.[14]

Perhaps not surprisingly, considering their increased exposure to medical trauma, people with a CHC have been found to be at significantly higher risk of developing PTSD. One study found that approximately 29% of adolescents who had undergone cardiac surgery as children were diagnosed with PTSD,[15] as compared to 5% of adolescents in the US general population,[16] while 11–21% of adults (with a CHC) had a diagnosis of PTSD compared to just 3.5% in the general population.[17] PTSD can also affect the wider family, with around a quarter of mothers and fathers experiencing acute PTSD 6 months after their child had undergone cardiac surgery.[18] It is perhaps not surprising to find this increased risk of developing PTSD in the CHC population, considering we are often exposed to the perfect storm of risk factors such as repeated, often unexpected, health crises and interventions while juggling additional life stressors often without adequate social support, which may result in what has been termed "cardiac disease–induced PTSD" (CDI-PTSD).[19]

This is concerning since it has been found that individuals with PTSD, especially when triggered by a medical trauma, are less likely to adhere to their prescribed medication regime. There are several reasons why this could be true; for many, taking medication serves as a reminder of the individual's original (medical) trauma.[20] Further, the relationship between the heart and PTSD is bidirectional, with studies reporting PTSD as a risk factor for heart disease, making it even more important that these difficulties are recognized and treated.[21]

Certain factors can increase our risk of developing a trauma disorder following exposure to a traumatic event, including feeling helpless and hopeless during the incident, poor social support during and following the incident, perceived life threat, an accumulation of traumatic events, other background life stressors, and pre-existing physical and mental health problems.[22] However, protective factors can improve mental health outcomes and help to mitigate the impact of psychological trauma, including adequate social support and help seeking,[23] being able to control some aspects of what is happening to you, feeling like you did the best you could during the event, being able to access appropriate psychological support,[24] and underlying "assumptions" about the benevolence of the world, the meaningfulness of events, and the worthiness of the self.[25]

Common Symptoms of Posttraumatic Stress Disorder

- Irritability or anger
- Nightmares or disturbing dreams of the traumatic event
- Tearfulness
- Anxiety
- Returning, upsetting memories about the event
- Insomnia
- Having a startle response, for instance jumping when you hear a loud noise or siren

- Going out of your way to avoid any exposure to the hospital or your care team
- Inability to concentrate

It is important to know that PTSD is a treatable condition and that help is available. You shouldn't have to live with these symptoms as they are very uncomfortable and intrusive. If you think you are experiencing this psychological condition it is essential that you speak to a healthcare professional.

Childhood Trauma

In his teens Andrew started to experience a lot of nightmares and flashbacks about earlier hospital experiences. He found they were often triggered by medical dramas on the TV or the smell of toast, which was the first thing he'd been given to eat after cardiac surgery as a child. He started to avoid these triggers but that became more and more tricky. Andrew spoke to his cardiology team, who referred him to a mental health professional. He was diagnosed with PTSD and offered therapy to help him process his traumatic medical experiences.

Chronic trauma can lead us to having a narrower window of tolerance and feeling less safe in our bodies, especially when we are exposed to such experiences during childhood. Throughout childhood, prolonged and chronic exposure to stressful and overwhelming events, especially in the absence of our main caregiver, can lead to structural changes within the brain that impact a child's ability to learn and to regulate emotions.[25]

The younger we are, the more vulnerable we are, given the increased dependency we have on our environment and the people within it to provide a sense of safety for us. Prior to the age of around 3 years, we do not store "episodic" memories of the events that happen to us. As such, we generally will be unable to recall our experiences as "stories." However, our body may store the memory of these traumatic events, shaping how safe we feel and how responsive we are to traumatic reminders and stressors. Although it may sound concerning to think that early trauma can change the brain, it is important to know that recovery also changes it. The main task of recovery for anyone subjected to traumatic childhood experiences is to find a way to feel safe in your body and to learn how to trust the messages your body is giving you.[26] We will cover strategies to this end in Chapters 5–7.

Other Types of Anxiety

Adults with CHCs have a higher probability of experiencing anxiety,[27] which can also present in other ways, including obsessive compulsive disorder (OCD), generalized anxiety disorder (GAD), and phobias (*DSM-5-TR*, 2013).[28]

Obsessive Compulsive Disorder

Obsessive compulsive disorder (OCD) is an anxiety disorder dominated by obsessive, intrusive thoughts or images that are followed by compulsive behaviors and rituals.[29] Often these obsessive thoughts center around hygiene, for example worry about becoming contaminated followed by obsessive hand washing. These thoughts can also present as "ego dystonic" thoughts (incompatible with the person's values) such as disturbing thoughts about causing harm to self or others, sexual thoughts, or about being inappropriate in public.

The thoughts associated with OCD cause a lot of distress. In fact, many people have these kinds of thoughts but are able to dismiss them easily. The difference with OCD is that the individual is deeply alarmed and often ashamed by them and engages in strategies to suppress them and compulsive behaviors to try and prevent or neutralize them. Such behaviors can be overt such as hand washing, switching plugs on and off, or reassurance seeking. They may also be mental rituals such as counting or replaying a situation over in your mind or looking for evidence of wrongdoing (sometimes called pure OCD). In the long term this reinforces the OCD cycle and perpetuates the problem. Having to perform increasingly complex rituals in response to these thoughts can become time-consuming and debilitating and can take over someone's life, impacting negatively on relationships, work, and productivity.

Often family members, in an attempt to relieve their loved one's distress, end up colluding with the problem by "helping" them carry out the OCD rituals or by repeatedly providing reassurance. Fear of losing control, intolerance of uncertainty, or a heightened sense of responsibility often underlies OCD, which can be triggered or exacerbated in response to a traumatic life event or by a major life transition (such as becoming a parent and worrying about keeping your new baby safe).

Exposure and response prevention therapy, a type of cognitive behavioral therapy (CBT), is an evidence-based treatment for OCD. While working with a therapist clients are encouraged to record their thoughts and behaviors and develop a hierarchy by ranking them in order of distress. Treatment generally involves gradually refraining from compulsive behaviors (or mental rituals) to break the OCD cycle and using anxiety management techniques to cope with distress (in place of the rituals). Therapy can also work to challenge and resolve any underlying issues such as a fear of losing control or heightened sense of responsibility.

Generalized Anxiety Disorder

Generalized anxiety disorder (GAD) is when an individual experiences excessive worry, more days than not, for at least 6 months about a wide range of situations and issues.[30] This debilitating condition also makes it difficult to control their worry and is often associated with a number of symptoms such as irritability, restlessness, trouble concentrating, physical symptoms of anxiety, and difficulty sleeping. Long-term health problems can increase vulnerability to GAD.[31]

Phobias

Anxiety disorders can also present as a phobia. A phobia is an overwhelming fear of a specific object, place, situation, feeling, or animal that is usually associated with a particular incident or trauma.[32] For example, a phobia of needles may develop following a difficult experience of having blood taken, or a social phobia may develop following workplace bullying. If a phobia becomes very severe, a person may organize their life around avoiding the thing that's causing them anxiety. This can restrict their day-to-day life and cause distress. Exposure therapy, a type of CBT, is an evidence-based treatment for phobias. Clients work with their therapist to develop an exposure hierarchy whereby they are gradually exposed to the stimuli that frighten them (e.g., in the case of a spider phobia, a photo of a spider, then a video of a spider, leading to eventually being in the same room as one), employing

anxiety management techniques to cope with distress and cognitive techniques to reframe and challenge any thoughts and beliefs that underlie the
phobia.

All of these anxiety disorders are treatable conditions. There are many
cognitive, behavioral, and emotional regulation strategies and techniques
that can help move us back into the window of tolerance when we notice
that we are activated. This is the place where we feel calm, safe, and clear
and better equipped to reach out for support, make good decisions, and be
present for the people that we care about. Controlled breathing, positive
imagery, and increased self-care are just a few tools that we will describe in
more detail in Chapters 5–7. Many people find therapy and/or medication
helpful to manage their anxiety. We will discuss tips for finding a therapist
in Chapter 10.

> *Once Jane started to recover from open heart surgery, she found going out in public
> really hard. She felt nervous that she might have a dizzy turn and worried that she
> might not be able to get back home quickly. Jane started to avoid going to places too far
> from home or where she knew she might bump into people. It just felt like too much
> having to answer their questions about how she was and what had happened. She knew
> they wouldn't understand and would make comments that would just annoy her. Over
> time Jane started to go out, at first when it was quiet and with a friend or relative, grad-
> ually building her confidence back up.*

Protective Factors and Posttraumatic Growth

The good news is that our response to difficult life events can be improved
by protective factors such as feeling good about how we responded (positive reframing), being able to access appropriate social support during and
afterward, feeling as safe as possible, feeling we are in control of at least some
aspects of what happened, and being able to access appropriate and timely
psychological support. We can even experience positive change following
adversity,[33] and we will discuss this more in Chapter 11. Mental health risk
and protective factors are summarized in Figure 3.5.

It is important to recognize that the reactions described earlier are very
common following stressful life events. They are not a sign of *weakness or
losing your mind*. You can begin to cope by making sense of what happened
(meaning-making); dealing with flashbacks and nightmares; addressing
sources of tension, irritability, and anger; reducing avoidance; improving

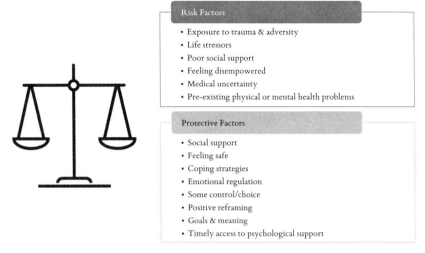

Figure 3.5 Mental health risk and protective factors. (Adapted from Porges 2011[6])

mood (mood management strategies); and improving the sleep–wake cycle. We will explore evidence-based techniques to help you manage anxiety in Chapters 5–7. By adopting a more trauma-informed approach, medical professionals can also play a role in helping to mitigate the impact of medically stressful events (see Chapter 12). Feeling empowered and informed about aspects of your medical care can also help (see Chapter 10).

4

Weathering the Storm

Low Mood, Shame, and Anger

Everyone experiences low mood occasionally, which may include sadness, anger, frustration, and irritability. It is normal to experience these feelings at times, especially when dealing with hardship or loss. Studies show that living with a congenital heart condition (CHC) can put us at a higher likelihood of experiencing bouts of low mood,[1] perhaps in direct response to the additional hardship and loss we can experience as a result of living with a CHC.

Often these feelings are a normal and understandable response to difficult life circumstances. The important thing is that we have support and strategies to get through the "hard times" because when these feelings are not dealt with they can lead to more serious mental health problems, such as depression. In this chapter we will explain the difference between a typical bout of feeling blue and the development of a more serious clinical depression. We will also discuss when and how we may want to seek additional support to help us to feel better. This is particularly important because of the established connection between depression, physical health, and heart conditions.

Some individuals with a CHC report feelings of helplessness, frustration, sadness, and anger when dealing with a new diagnosis, cardiac symptoms, or simply when reflecting on the impact of their health. They may feel resentful of others who seem to breeze through life without having to deal with the same difficulties. As described, these feelings to a certain extent are a normal response. Perhaps there is a sadness associated with an inability to participate in a physical activity you once enjoyed or always hoped to, or a sense of helplessness regarding multiple hospitalizations or foreboding about what the future may hold. You may also be disappointed about being unable to take part in something your peers are able to take for granted, or you may feel angry about a decline in your health. Finding healthy ways to express and process these feelings is important for your emotional health and well-being.

Sometimes we develop less healthy coping strategies to deal with these disappointments, such as social withdrawal, dependency on alcohol, over-eating or undereating, taking drugs, or trying to overcompensate by push-ing ourselves really hard and being self-critical. Or we may learn to suppress these difficult feelings by pushing them away, and then find ourselves suf-fering from panic attacks, depression, or unexplained physical symptoms seemingly out of the blue.

It is essential that we learn to recognize our normal response to the life events we face and find healthy ways to process and manage these feelings to protect our mental health and well-being and enable us to live as fully as possible.

Veil of Silence

There are many factors that can get in the way of us being able to recognize and process distressing feelings. For the most part the unique challenges that we face as a result of having a CHC are not shared by our family and peers, and in most situations, society just isn't designed to accommodate people with lifelong cardiac issues. Because of this, it can be difficult to get valid-ation for what we are feeling, and often we have to find ways to navigate these feelings by ourselves. It can be easy to forget this and wonder why we are struggling with other more typical life issues when those around us are not. The fact that our family and peers are not experiencing these issues can mean that we minimize their impact on us. Because there is no one to share them with, no common language or representation in films, TV shows, or books, we may "compare and despair" if we fall behind in our education or life goals or are unable to "keep up" with our peers. It is essential we recog-nize this and stop comparing ourselves to others who are on a completely different life journey.

We might even become self-critical, attributing our distress to some-thing wrong with us rather than acknowledging the hidden barriers that even we don't see. It is important to recognize these additional challenges and the feelings they evoke so that you can validate your lived experience and accommodate any additional support, time, or understanding you may need and deserve. We will talk more about this in Chapters 5–9.

Expressing your feelings, or emotional release, is essential to your overall health and well-being. Usually it feels good to have the opportunity to get it off your chest. Some of us may have picked up on messages from early on that we should be brave and grateful for the life we have been gifted and that by showing our distress or vulnerability we are somehow disrespecting our care providers, upsetting our family, or being a burden. We may even feel that showing emotion makes us weak. Expressing a normal response to difficult life events is not weak. Quite the opposite: showing vulnerability takes courage. This is not disrespectful to anyone, and it does not mean that you are ungrateful. Sharing your feelings and asking for support means that you are strong and moving toward positive change. Social support is one of the most protective factors for mental health and well-being, and it is essential that we are able to access this.

There can also be a wider cultural veil of silence within the CHC community where individuals are reluctant to share their experiences because they don't want to seem like "a complainer," attract pity, worry their loved ones, or feel they need to shield their stories from parents with newly diagnosed children or others with the same condition. Of course, we don't want to upset anyone, and there is always an appropriate time and place for sharing our experiences. Yet it is important to find a supportive place where you are able to safely tell and share your story, especially the difficult parts. This will hopefully enable you to feel a sense of relief and to integrate your lived experiences. Further, lessons can't be learned unless we share, discuss, and work together to make things better.

Because we live with our heart condition for our entire lives, ironically we don't always get the same support that others do when they develop a medical condition. It is taken for granted that someone who has been newly diagnosed with cancer or an acquired heart problem will have an emotional and psychological reaction to this. It is routinely accepted that they will need support throughout their sometimes time-limited treatment and medical journey, with holistic care packages often being offered. Yet we (and others) often don't recognize this need across our own CHC lifelong journey, somehow expecting ourselves to remain stoic regardless of the many bumps along the road.

Sometimes we don't feel these responses during the triggering situation because we go into survival mode. For example, if you are told during a routine hospital checkup that you need to stay in the hospital for further tests, you may appear to cope well with this news. You might jump into autopilot and organize your work and family, arrange a hospital bag, and figure out all the practical logistics. You might make jokes with your care team and family "Here we go again" or "I just like to keep life interesting." It may be after the storm has passed, once you are recovering back at home, that you start to feel upset. This is entirely normal. Often our bodies go into survival mode in response to threat and adversity. Often it is only afterward, when we feel safe again, that we start to process these feelings.

Grief and Loss

> *Grief and resilience live together.*
>
> —Michelle Obama, *Becoming*[2]

When most people hear the terms *grief* and *bereavement*, they usually think of feelings related to the death of a loved one. However, bereavement is the anguish experienced after significant loss, and this can also be relevant to individuals (and family members) in the CHC community. Many of us have suffered significant losses as a result of our CHC. Some of these losses may be hard to recognize because they involve the loss of something we never knew, such as a "normal" childhood, missing out on activities others can take for granted, rejection because of our perceived differences, and missed work or social opportunities. Some of us face finding out we are unable to have children or are unable to have as big a family as we had hoped. We may face a significant decline in health status, or we may have the realization that we may not have the energy or stamina to do some of the activities that we always enjoyed. For some, the feelings of loss are tied up with the knowledge that at some point they will need to have another surgery or are at high risk for a sudden traumatic medical event. Some examples include concerns about when a heart valve might need to be repaired or replaced and if a heart transplant will be needed in the future. Learning to live with an implantable cardiac device and dealing with possible shocks from their implantable cardioverter-defibrillator (ICD) and future battery and lead replacements are also worries we hear about. Many individuals are grieving the reality of their lifelong health situation, and this is understandable.

It is important to know that feeling sad is a completely normal response to loss. Some other ways grief is experienced or expressed are listed in Table 4.1.

Feelings of grief can sometimes be complicated by society's reaction to these feelings.[3] For example, many assume that the longer one lives with a loss, or if they had suffered similar losses before, they will adapt or recover better. Sometimes others assume "since they have lived with this their entire life, they should be over it by now" or "they've been through this before so they are more equipped to handle it" or "they don't know any difference anyway." Reactions such as these can make it more difficult for individuals to recognize, acknowledge, and understand their feelings of grief.

Once we are able to link our experiences to our feelings, then the real healing can begin. This usually takes time, so it is important to give yourself the space that you need to process when these feelings began and what may have triggered them. During this time, it is important to allow yourself to experience a full range of emotions. It is normal to feel sad, scared, or angry as a result of a loss. We suggest finding someone you trust to talk to about these feelings. If it isn't possible to speak with family or friends, there are a number of peer support groups that many individuals find helpful. Your healthcare team might be able to refer you to one, and if not there are a number of online peer support groups. We have listed resources in the

Table 4.1 Stages of Grief

Disbelief	"They must have gotten the diagnosis wrong!"
Denial	"I'm sure it's not that serious. I don't have any new symptoms."
Guilt	"I shouldn't have pushed myself so hard."
Despair	"I can't deal with this." "I don't think I can handle it."
Anger	"Why does this keep happening to me?" "Just leave me alone!"
Bargaining	"If I follow my doctor's orders and continue to be a good person, this will get better."
Acceptance	"This is my new reality and I have to focus on what I *can* do and make a new plan."
Finding meaning	"How can I grow around my grief?" "What can I do and who will I become?" "How can I redefine myself?"

Appendix. In some cases, locating an experienced mental health professional can be very helpful as well.

It is important to know that after a loss, in time, it is quite possible to rebuild and find new meaning in life. But it is not simply time that helps us to heal; it is also what you do with that time that is important. Trying to numb the pain with distraction, alcohol, or drugs will only complicate the healing process. Part of finding that meaning is making sure that you find the support and receive validation for your pain and experiences. During this time, it is important that you are gentle with yourself by paying attention to all of your needs. This includes taking care of yourself physically, emotionally, socially, and spiritually. It will ultimately mean accepting that things may have changed, but holding the knowledge that it is possible to find new sources of joy, happiness, and meaning in your life. We personally know many individuals with a CHC who have accomplished this. They have gotten support, grieved in a healthy way, and created a beautiful life that is inspiring to so many.

Denial is a common defense mechanism when experiencing a loss. It is a strategy that individuals use to protect themselves from the reality of a situation, and it helps them to reduce anxiety. It allows them to take time to subconsciously process, integrate, and adjust to the news at their own pace. While this is a normal, short-term response, it becomes problematic when it is prolonged and begins to affect the way you take care of yourself physically and get the help that you need. Here are some examples:

> *Maggie is an 18-year-old who moved into college for the first time. She has been through several surgeries due to her CHC and wants to put "the hard times behind me." She strives to "be normal" even if it means drinking alcohol excessively and smoking marijuana with her peers.*

> *Dan is a 32-year-old attorney who just started his new job in a big firm. He has a CHC and has had a pacemaker since childhood. He is proud of his recent professional accomplishments and doesn't want anything to get in the way of his success. He has been having a lot of heart palpitations and dizzy spells but avoids going in to see his adult congenital heart disease doctor. He says he keeps "forgetting" but deep down may avoid calling for fear of being told he must return to the hospital. Dan tells himself "these symptoms are probably just the excitement and stress of starting a new job."*

There is some evidence that suggests that denial is used more frequently in individuals with a CHC.[4] Denial is often associated with depression and anxiety and may impede an individual's ability to adhere to doctor's recommendations, develop healthy life choices, and recognize that they need more support. This is concerning because these are all essential aspects of living a healthy lifestyle, thriving, and reaching one's fullest potential, both physically and psychologically.

Recognizing Depression

Depression is more than low mood or a normative reaction to loss. It is a serious mental health condition that merits specialist treatment. Without proper treatment it can be a life-threatening illness. Many studies suggest there is a real link between depression and one's physical health, particularly when it comes to heart disease. Specifically, depressed individuals tend to be less likely to follow doctor's orders, take their medications, eat a heart-healthy diet, and follow recommendations for physical activity.[5] Another study reports that there is evidence that depression is a risk factor for having additional cardiac events.[6] While this study focused on patients with coronary artery disease, it is likely to be relevant for all cardiac patients, highlighting the importance of recognizing and accessing prompt treatment for depression.

Red Flag Signs and Symptoms of Depression

- Loss of interest in activities you used to enjoy
- Withdrawing from family and friends
- Lack of concentration
- Feeling overwhelmed, indecisive
- Loss of confidence and low self-worth
- Increased alcohol, drug use, and/or vaping or smoking
- Sleep problems (sleeping too much or too little)
- Feeling helpless, worthless, and guilty
- Increased irritability, anger, mood swings
- Feeling sad most of the time
- Inappropriate or excessive guilt
- Negative or depressed thinking
- Suicidal thoughts or self-harming behaviors

If you recognize these signs and symptoms and they have been present every day for at least 2 weeks,[7] it is important that you speak to a care provider and seek professional support.

Depression: Nature versus Nurture

There are a lot of different reasons why someone may develop depression. Depression is a serious mood disorder that results from a complex interplay among social, psychological, and biological factors that requires assessment, diagnosis, and treatment from a qualified mental health professional.[8] Sometimes individuals report feeling depressed "for no apparent reason," often "out of the blue," and feel confused about why they are feeling low. Often this is the result of a gradual accumulation of stressors, leaving it hard to pinpoint a single trigger. Sometimes depression is a result of being strong for too long, and it can be our body's way of telling us we need to take some time out to focus on recovery, recuperation, and self-care.

Genetic factors can increase our vulnerability to depression, and as such it is important to get a history of mental health issues in the family. Mental healthcare providers will consider this to be an important part of your mental health assessment.

Underlying physical health problems can also contribute to depression, including hormonal conditions such as hypothyroidism (also known as an underactive thyroid), autoimmune conditions and inflammatory markers,[9] alcohol and drug abuse, sleep apnea, and certain medications. Natural hormonal changes associated with the menstrual cycle, menopause, and pregnancy can also increase risk. For others, there may be some underlying neurological factors, influencing the concentration of "chemical messengers" or neurotransmitters in our brains and hormone levels.[10] Seasonal affective disorder (SAD) can also increase risk due to a lack of Vitamin D during the dark winter months.

The good news is that depression is treatable and even curable. Depression is commonly treated with psychotherapy, medication, or a combination of both. There is no one-size-fits-all fix, and often it is about finding what approach works best for you individually. Once your depression lifts, so do your increased risks.[11]

Anger and Resentment

Anger is also a normal response to adversity. We feel angry when something is unfair, and this can motivate us to address any injustice. There are many understandable reasons why some of us with a CHC may feel angry in re-sponse to the unfairness of being born with a serious, lifelong medical con-dition, possibly missing out, facing invasive hospital procedures that no one else in your peer group does, and facing additional obstacles in life such as discrimination. Recognizing this feeling, identifying the reasons for it, and finding healthy ways to express it are important.

Anger is an "activating" emotion quite similar to anxiety because our body is preparing for defense (it is the fight in the fight/flight response). In response we may feel hot and sweaty, our heart may start racing, while our breathing becomes more rapid, our legs might feel weak, and we may feel shaky. Our judgment may become impaired, and we may get the urge to act impulsively. Sometimes resentments can occur, relation-ships can be negatively affected, or we may end up feeling humiliated. It is important to recognize the initial signs of anger, which makes it easier to step back, calm yourself, and shift your thinking to avoid behaving in a way you may later regret (we will cover techniques to manage anger in Chapters 5–7).

It is completely natural, at times, to feel resentment toward other who do not have to deal with the same load as you. These may include peers, sib-lings, colleagues, or healthcare providers who can take their health privilege for granted. Without shared experience they may make flippant comments such as "But you look well," "You are just attention seeking," or "You just use your condition when it suits you" or invalidate the challenges you face, for example by comparing your experience of open heart surgery with that time they had their tonsils removed!

Similarly, envy is an emotion that can fester and grow. Some individuals, with or without a CHC, feel envious at times. Many societies contribute to this envy by messaging the value of "having more" and "doing more." Social media can perpetuate this with accounts full of smiling, healthy-looking friends on amazing adventures. As an individual with a CHC, you may have been envious of your friends' or family members' physical abil-ities, carefree attitude about their good health, and ability to attend school or their job without health-related interruptions. It is important to know that what you see or what a person portrays is not always the true picture. Most people have struggles of their own whether they let us know about them or not. Try not to allow yourself to make assumptions that you are the only one struggling, and try to meditate on accepting these differences and work on rooting for the individual/s and sharing in their good fortune.

Sometimes we can be angry about something but not recognize it consciously. This can occasionally happen to people who have suffered from a traumatic event. If this connection is not made, the anger can sometimes "leak out" in other unrelated areas of your life. Some of the ways it can come is through cynical, self-deprecating, or passive-aggressive behaviors. These behaviors can affect your mood, relationships, and your overall health and quality of life. Regardless of the root of your anger, it is important to learn to deal with it in a healthy way. If not, it can become self-destructive, negatively affecting your relationships and your overall physical health; unprocessed anger "turned inward" can lead to self-criticism, feeling helpless, and depression.

The problem is that when we feel angry we are often not in the best place to communicate effectively. Even if we have a legitimate reason for our anger, if we communicate this aggressively, we are unlikely to get our needs met. It is important to note that anger and aggression are not the same. Anger is often a legitimate emotion in response to what has happened to you. Aggression is a communication style when we try to dominate another person and impose our own needs over theirs. We will go into this in more detail in Chapter 8. When feeling angry, it is important to take some time out to calm down, think about what you want to communicate, and then return to the situation when you feel calmer. The goal in expressing your anger is to avoid being aggressive or passive and when ready to communicate to do it in a calm but assertive way.

Self-pity can be another emotional "trap." Life is hard, and for some of us with a CHC, it can be even harder. It is understandable to wonder why something is happening, feel it is unfair (it is!), and to feel badly about it. You may even ask, "Why me?" However, we want to be careful not to become overly focused on the negative aspects of our lives. Acknowledgment is important, but we need to accept what we cannot change and look forward. Sometimes this means picking up where we left off (before the difficult event), or it may mean figuring out a new plan to move forward, which sometimes requires us to redefine ourselves (we will discuss goal setting in Chapter 10) because if a CHC teaches us anything it is how very precious life is.

Of course, often we can't do anything about some of the things we may feel angry about, such as being born with a CHC. The reality is that life is often unfair. Some of us are dealt a worse hand than others. It is okay to acknowledge this. It is important to not get "stuck" on this because you will only make life even harder for yourself. If this is the case, it can help to find outlets for this anger, such as writing it down, speaking to someone, or seeking therapy. It can also help to channel this energy into something productive such as a passion for music, painting, gardening, or whatever your interest might be. Creating meaning from our experiences is also therapeutic such as getting involved in advocacy work, raising funds for a charity you support, or offering peer mentorship for others with a CHC such as younger people coming up. Acceptance and shifting your focus to what you can do is key to living well with whatever life throws at you. You likely know better than most how to live well with the hand you have been dealt! We will cover more on the topic of anger and aggression in Chapters 6–8.

Shame and Guilt

Guilt and shame are two different negative, self-reflective emotions which sometimes can occur together. It is very easy to get the two emotions confused; however, they are a bit different. Shame is usually felt when a person believes they are unable to be their perceived ideal self, due to circumstances out of our control.[12] This is when we feel embarrassed or humiliated about the perception that something is wrong about us, that we are fundamentally bad or defective *as a person.* Guilt, on the other hand, is connected to something we feel we have done wrong or something we are responsible for. In other words, guilt is usually directed toward the action and shame is directed toward the self. In terms of how this affects our behavior, guilt can prompt us to apologize or make reparations, and shame can cause us to withdraw, criticize ourselves, or engage in self-punitive behaviors.

Guilt can actually sometimes be healthy if we learn from it and remedy a wrong. If we say something hurtful to someone, guilt can prompt us to apologize for our insensitive actions or prompt us to change behaviors that are harmful to ourselves. Guilt can also be unhealthy when blaming yourself for something you cannot control. Some examples of unhealthy guilt include the following:

- Feeling guilty about your fatigue
- Feeling guilty that you are no longer able to work
- Feeling guilty about the impact your CHC has on your family

As social animals, it is normal to feel shame when we feel left out or are made to feel different. Shame is a debilitating emotion that we feel in response to a "social threat," activating our *fight, flight, or freeze response*. As social beings, we have evolved to feel safer when we are included in the social group. If we do not feel included, we can feel shame, wanting to disappear or hide away for our own self-protection. We also become very self-conscious and may feel helpless and powerless or angry.[13] If we feel shame regularly, it can have a detrimental impact on our self-esteem and lead to depression and possibly even self-harming behaviors.

Self-criticism is a common symptom of shame. We may berate ourselves with statements such as "You are not good enough," "You're a failure," or "You are weak." Often the self-criticism is internalized from a real experience we have encountered with an abuser, bully, critical parent, caregiver, teacher, or unrealistic social expectations. We may have internalized any discrimination we have experienced about "being different." This may have been overt, but sometimes it originates from what didn't happen such as a lack of social inclusion or representation in public life, the media, and arts.[14]

Shame can lead to us to reject parts of ourselves (such as our health condition) and overcompensate by setting unrealistically high standards. When we fail to meet the unrealistically high bar we set ourselves, we use this as further evidence that we "aren't good enough," reinforcing this unhelpful belief. We may engage in punitive behaviors such as perfectionism or risky behaviors and not look after our health (see Figure 4.1).

It is helpful to talk about feeling different, shame, and low self-confidence. Shame thrives and grows in the dark; throw light on it and it will shrink and die. If you are experiencing any of these feelings, please know that they can be worked through. If these feelings aren't recognized and talked about, they can lead to anger, resentment, low self-worth, and even clinical depression.

We will explore more about how to overcome the "self-critic" and develop self-compassion in Chapter 8. If any of this sounds familiar to you, it

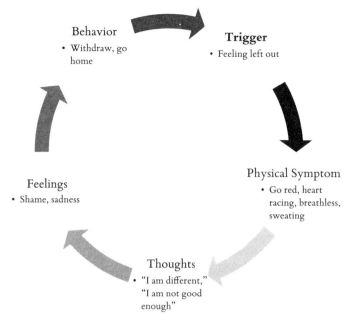

Figure 4.1 Shame vicious cycle.

may be time for you to make a plan to address these feelings. We will discuss more about when to seek further support and Mental Health: Red Flag Symptoms at the end of Chapter 7.

5

Self-Care and Stress Management Toolkit

Since those of us navigating life with a congenital heart condition (CHC) can face unique, additional stressors throughout life; it is even more important for us to take care of ourselves, establish a toolkit of coping strategies, and build a strong network of social support. Over the next four chapters we will outline the most recent evidence-based strategies to help you reduce background stress, understand and manage your emotions, tackle any unhelpful behaviors and thinking styles, and establish a strong support team. Many of these strategies may be equally useful to loved ones and caregivers.

Developing a toolkit of techniques and strategies to help you manage any distressing feelings that are triggered by your health-related experiences (or everyday stressors!) is essential to combating stress and handling difficult emotions. Furthermore, proactively reducing background stress and enhancing feelings of calm and relaxation can also help tremendously. There are a wide range of evidence-based techniques that have been shown to be effective; however, it is important to note that different techniques work for different people, depending on the issue and the timing. We recommend that you experiment with some of these techniques to explore what works for you.

Reduce Your Baseline Stress

Proactively working to calm your baseline stress levels makes it easier to stay in the window of tolerance when you face challenging situations (described in Chapter 3). When you are in a calmer frame of mind, it will be less likely for your alarm response to switch you into fight, flight, or freeze. This is because an accumulation of stress over time can make us more ready to quickly switch into our alarm response. By proactively reducing your baseline stress with self-care, you can mitigate against any stressors you can't control. If you try to keep your baseline stress low, it takes a significant life event for you to reach the threshold for fight, flight, or freeze. If you have an accumulation of a lot of stressful factors, it doesn't take much for the alarm to go off (any small thing may be "the final straw"). This is why self-care and proactively working to reduce your baseline stress levels is so essential. There are many different ways you can do this, and we have described some techniques here.

Self-Care

Self-care is fundamental to reducing baseline stress levels and building resilience.[1] Caring for yourself is an essential part of feeling well both emotionally and physically. Taking some time out gives you the chance to "reset and restore." Just as we all have physical hygiene habits (brushing our teeth, clipping our nails), we also need to develop habits for a healthy mind, sometimes called mental hygiene. The key is to incorporate the tools you find to be helpful into your daily routine so they can become a habit. Self-care includes maintaining a healthy sleep routine, eating well, mindfulness, and moving your body on a daily basis. Sometimes self-care means treating yourself to a nice dinner, scheduling a massage, or taking a few days off from work when you need some extra TLC. However, more than this, self-care involves being compassionate to yourself, especially regarding any limitations or difficulties you face because of your health condition and setting appropriate boundaries in relationships (described in Chapter 8). The most important relationship you have is with yourself. Therefore, we all need to treat ourselves with great care, just as we would treat a valued friend or family member. It can be helpful to schedule this time into your calendar or make yourself more accountable by telling someone your plan.

The Importance of Sleep

Sound sleep is one of the best gifts you can give yourself. Deep sleep helps us to heal, and it is essential to growth, health, and general well-being. Not getting enough sleep or sleeping too much is a common complaint for many adults, and this can not only lead to feeling tired the following day, but it can also decrease your body's ability to fight off illnesses and it can negatively affect your mood. Sleeping too much (hypersomnia) may also be a symptom of depression and can also interfere with day-to-day life.

It is helpful to determine how much sleep you need; while 8 hours is the average, this may vary significantly from person to person. There is no point forcing yourself to try and sleep for 8 hours if you only need 6; likewise if you still feel tired after getting a full 8 hours of sleep, you may need more. The amount of sleep we need can also change over time with age, activity levels, and stress.

While everyone has occasional sleep disruptions, if sleeplessness becomes more of a rule rather than an exception, it may be time to give it some of your attention. Insomnia, frequent waking, and hypersomnia are sometimes caused by a simple shift in your schedule, dietary change, or life stressor. As soon as these changes or stressors are modified, regular sleep often resumes. Sometimes sleep disturbance is caused by poor sleep habits. Sleep hygiene is a set of healthy behaviors that become a routine which we engage in leading up to bedtime. Just as we foster personal hygiene habits (shower, brushing teeth, etc.), we need to also create and follow a set of habits that foster a healthy sleep cycle.

If you are having difficulty sleeping and can't identify why, a sleep journal may help. Keep it up for 2 weeks and then evaluate your habits. Paying attention to your sleep hygiene is one of the most important things you can do to maintain good sleep.[2]

Sleep Hygiene Tips

- Try to go to bed the same time each night and get up at the same time each morning.
- Make sure your bedroom is dark enough; install blackout blinds, if needed.

- Keep the bedroom quiet when sleeping.
- Use your bed only for sleep and for sex.
- Try to eat your last big meal at least 3 hours before bedtime.
- Keep an eye on alcohol consumption as it can disrupt your natural sleep cycle.
- Avoid caffeine (including hidden caffeine, e.g., in soft drinks) and sugar in the evenings.
- Create a relaxing routine each night and repeat (cup of decaf tea, bath, reading, stretching).
- Get regular physical activity each day.
- Get regular exposure to outdoor light.
- Try guided meditation or other relaxation exercises before going to sleep.

Sleep Tips: What to Avoid

- Caffeine in the late afternoon and evening.
- Daytime naps.
- Excessive television, Internet use, or mobile phone scrolling at night.
- Stimulating activity just before bed (scary movie, emotional discussion).
- The use of alcohol or nonprescription drugs to get to sleep.
- Eating a big meal right before you sleep.
- Taking another person's sleeping pills.
- Taking over-the-counter sleep medication, unless your doctor suggests it.

It can help to determine a time of the night to wind down. This is a time that you close the kitchen, your phone, and other electronics to begin to prepare your body for the treasured time of the day to just rest and re-juvenate. You may need to replace a habit with a new one, for instance listening to calming music instead of watching the news or connecting to a free guided imagery meditation app instead of scrolling through social media. Once it's time for lights out, don't allow yourself to lie in bed awake for more than 30 minutes. If that happens, get up and engage in a quiet activity such as reading a book or journaling. When you begin to feel sleepy, return to bed. Repeat this as many times as necessary. Give it time. It can take up to 2 weeks to reset your sleep cycle, so don't despair if this doesn't work after the first few nights.

If there aren't any clear-cut reasons for your sleep difficulty and you are practicing sound sleep hygiene, it could also be a symptom of something physical such as hormonal changes, medication side effects, an underlying illness, or mental health issues. In this case, we recommend that you see your primary care physician to rule out certain illnesses. If sleep apnea is suspected, your physician may refer you to a sleep center.

If all physical reasons are ruled out, then it may be time to consider exploring any underlying stress or mental health issues. Insomnia or hypersomnia can be caused by anxiety or depression. Sometimes sleep problems begin in direct response to a stressful life, but they become maintained, even after the stressor has resolved, by a conditioned, emotional response in the way you think about your sleep. Your thoughts and behaviors surrounding your sleep problem ("I'm going to be so tired tomorrow!" or "I will be up all night" or clock watching until the alarm goes off) could be making it worse. A mental health practitioner can evaluate and help with any of these contributing factors. Cognitive behavioral therapy, stress management strategies, and mindfulness/relaxation exercises can often help to get individuals back on track with healthy sleep. Occasionally a referral may be made to a psychiatrist for a medication consultation. If a medication is prescribed, it is best if the psychiatrist works together with your therapist for a combined treatment approach.

Poor sleep quality is not something to ignore. Very often it can be improved with increased insight and basic shifts in schedule or habits. Once your sleep cycle is back on track, you will hopefully begin to feel better and have more energy, which will help to improve your overall health and quality of life.

Diet and Exercise

What we eat and our physical activity can make a huge difference to how we feel physically, emotionally, and psychologically. In terms of nutrition, we suggest speaking with your adult congenital heart disease (ACHD) specialist to check to see if there are any dietary modifications that need to be made. For instance, some individuals with a CHC feel better on a low-sodium diet, and for others caffeine and/or alcohol may need to be cut back or avoided. Generally speaking, large amounts of alcohol can cause your heart to beat rapidly or abnormally, and it can increase the risk of blood clots, so it is best to avoid binge drinking.[3]

What we eat directly affects our mood. In fact, 60% of the dry weight of the brain is made up of unsaturated fats, which are found in nuts, seeds, olives, oily fish, rapeseed, and vegetable oils; you literally are what you eat. Plenty of fruits and vegetables and whole-grain cereal foods, with some protein foods, including fatty fish, will support a good supply of nutrients for good health and good mood.[4] Eating regular meals that consist of slow energy-release foods also helps our body by maintaining our blood-sugar levels and keeping our energy levels consistent. It is important to bear in mind that caffeine and stimulant (energy) drinks can have an effect on the heart as they can cause an instant rise in blood pressure and heart rate.

Gut health is also increasingly being linked to mood. If you have been prescribed antibiotics for infection or post-surgery, you may benefit from taking a course of probiotics to maintain a healthy gut. Again this is something you should discuss with your healthcare team. Some people find meeting with a registered dietician or nutritionist helpful in coming up with ideas for healthy meal plans. Maintaining a healthy weight will put less pressure on your heart and improve your general well-being.

> *I hated sports growing up. I was always the slowest kid in gym class, and because I don't look like I have anything wrong with me, I got made fun of a lot. I've never felt confident about my physical abilities because of that. It took me a long time as an adult to get used to the idea of having a morning work out routine, instead of just avoiding physical activity altogether. I still won't workout at a gym, but do YouTube workouts at home.*
>
> —Lenae, 33 years old, United States

The majority of people born with heart problems can lead a full and active life and do not need to restrict their physical activity. Studies show that for many, exercise can be as effective as taking an antidepressant medication to lessen symptoms of depression.[5] For some individuals with a CHC, exercise isn't always that straightforward. In the early days many of us were told that we should not exercise at all. Recommendations from healthcare providers to restrict physical activity were common for many years. We may have been told to sit out during gym classes at school or struggled to keep up with our peers. These recommendations have changed significantly over the years, and the importance of physical activity for healthy heart and general health is now widely recognized.[6] Likewise, the damaging effect of physical inactivity and obesity on health means that exercising, within your own personal safe limits, is often recommended.

I have always been jealous of the physical activity that my peers can complete. Things changed when my arrhythmia was cured by a catheter ablation. After that I was able to increase the intensity of my walks and my football became more physical. I decided to try and visit 45 peaks over 450 meters; the highest point I reached was 890 meters. I felt a great sense of pride in completing the challenge, but it was tinged with regret for the years of physical fitness that I'd missed due to my CHDs and psychological challenges.
—*Zeb, 55 years old, United Kingdom*

Yet psychologically exercise may be a struggle if you have grown up feeling fearful of "pushing" yourself physically or you have missed out on the experience of learning your own physical limits. This is completely understandable, and if this is the case, it might take some time to build up your confidence. It might help to start small, for example by going for walks, and building yourself up (within the parameters agreed upon by your cardiac team). On the other hand, some people may have gotten different messages growing up and enjoy defying the odds by training and pushing their bodies (i.e., signing up for running events).

I find maintaining a level of fitness challenging. Some activities are harder than others, particularly those which require greater cardiovascular activity. Often, I feel like I can't keep up with exercise and physical activities that my friends can do with ease. As my heartbeat increases with exercise, I worry about overexertion and my heart not coping with even moderate amounts of exercise. This hesitation and overcautious approach in turn impacts reaching and maintaining an appropriate level of fitness.
—*Benjamin, 39 years old, Australia*

Regardless of your personal goals, we always suggest speaking with your ACHD specialist about what level of exercise you can do safely. Your cardiologist might order some tests before making a recommendation, which may include an echocardiogram or cardiopulmonary stress test. The stress test usually involves taking part in graded exercise, such as walking on a running machine, while your heart is being monitored so that your team can monitor how well your heart and lungs work during exertion as your physical activity level increases.

Once a recommendation is made, they may be able to give you an exercise prescription which will outline the parameters and their suggestions. There is a wide range of physical activity that may be recommended, from simple stretching to, chair yoga to finding an enjoyable low- or high-impact cardiovascular workout.

If you have a pacemaker or cardiac device and you are struggling with exertion, it may be useful to ask your cardiac physiology team to review the settings on your device to ensure they are optimal for you. This may involve taking part in a cardiopulmonary stress test.

You may be able to access a cardiac rehabilitation program as part of your healthcare team, either post cardiac surgery or if you would like to learn more about what exercise would work for you. This may include access to a specialist physiotherapist who can help you establish an exercise program tailored to your health condition and status.

A fitness tracker or a walking app can also be a helpful way to increase your physical activity levels. This can also provide useful information about your heart rate that you can monitor to make sure you are staying within the limits recommended by your cardiology team. Some smartwatches can measure your heart rate and alert you if your sustained heart rate goes above a threshold value. Some can even record an electrocardiogram that you can share with your doctor to pinpoint what kind of heart rhythm is associated with, for example, a rapid heart rate. This can be particularly useful if you are having unexplained episodes of palpitations or dizziness. Modern pacemakers can also communicate with home tracking devices that can send reports to your cardiac team remotely. If you have a pace-maker or implantable cardioverter-defibrillator (ICD), be sure to check with your electrophysiologist to be sure any tracking device doesn't inter-fere with your device.

Some General Lifestyle Tips

Some people with a CHC find that they are less able to tolerate very hot or very cold weather. It can help to stay in the shade or somewhere that has air conditioning if it is too hot and humid. Prolonged exposure to the sun is best avoided. Extra care may be necessary with some medica-tion, for example amiodarone, which can make the skin more sensitive to sunlight.

Being prepared and making sure you have lots of layers of clothing can help when it is cold. If you have circulation problems, then you may feel colder during the night. Taking a hot water bottle to bed, using a heated blanket (if you have a pacemaker or ICD, make sure it is compatible), wrapping up, and wearing bed socks may help. Some people with a CHC report dehydrating more easily, too, so making sure you keep hydrated is also wise.

Good hygiene practices such as regularly washing your hands; using hand gel; staying away from people who have a virus, a cough, or runny nose; keeping yourself warm; and making sure you get your annual flu vaccine are important for everyone. Studies have also indicated the importance of good oral hygiene for good heart health to prevent infective endocarditis. Taking care of your teeth and gums is important, and for some individuals prophylctic antibiotics may be indicated prior to any invasive dental treatments.[7] Other factors that may risk blood infection and endocarditis, such as getting a tattoo or piercing, are also cautioned against by care providers; again this is something to discuss with your healthcare team.

There may be some restrictions on activities depending on your CHC condition and whether you have a cardiac device. For example, for some devices it is recommended that you avoid strong magnets and do not pass through metal detectors (e.g., security at the airport). Bungee jumping, for example, is not recommended for people on warfarin or for those who have an electrical device implanted. It is important to be aware that traveling to areas of high altitude can also have an effect on the cardiovascular system. Some people with a CHC may want to scuba dive, ski, or parachute jump, but it is sensible to fully understand the risks first by discussing with your cardiologist or ACHD nurse specialist.

It is important to note that saunas and heated spa pools can lower your blood pressure and increase your heart rate, so follow medical advice for your condition regarding the length of time you may safely stay in them.[8]

Schedule Pleasant and Relaxing Events

To experience good mental health and well-being, we need to make sure that we are experiencing joy and pleasure in our lives. Sometimes work, chores, and obligations take over, and we forget to look after ourselves. However, it is really important that we experience a balance of rewarding, enjoyable experiences to maintain our health and well-being and to reduce stress. It can be useful to schedule events to look forward to (going on a holiday), shorter-term treats (going for a meal or meeting a friend), and smaller experiences that we can fit into the corners of the day (reading a book or listening to music).

Clearly we all find different things enjoyable and relaxing. We have included some suggestions here, but there may be others and we encourage you to make a list of your own. Think about what brings you joy; this may include activities you enjoyed when you were younger but have long since stopped doing.

Relaxing Activities

- Crafting, painting, drawing, or do-it-yourself projects
- Listening to music, singing, or dancing
- Reading or listening to an audio book or podcast
- Exercising: going for a swim, cycling, or visiting the gym
- Going for a massage
- Going for a drive
- Having a long bath or shower
- Planning a trip
- Cooking or baking
- Gardening
- "Forest bathing," or immersing yourself in a green space
- Gaming (computer)
- Writing, journaling, or blogging
- Meeting, calling, or messaging a friend or family member
- Playing a musical instrument
- Stretching

Build Your Resilience

Resilience is the process and the ability to overcome hardship, trauma, or significant stress. It is how well we can bounce back emotionally when something difficult happens to us. It is resilience that helps protect us from getting too overwhelmed by life's challenges. Resilience can be preserved and, with effort, can even be increased. It takes attention and insight into your thoughts and behaviors to positively affect your ability to withstand adversity. It is about choosing thoughts and interpreting life's challenges in a way that is truthful, but always considering the narrative that helps you to become more positive, grateful, hopeful, and strong.

Preserve and Build upon Your Resilience

- Surround yourself with supportive and positive people.
- Limit the time you spend watching or listening to stressful news programs.
- Turn off any news alerts you may have set on your electronic devices.
- Do not overschedule yourself.
- Learn to say no.
- Limit your social media screen time (especially "compare and despair" content).
- Get physical in a safe way.
- Get outside and connect with nature whenever possible.
- Become more mindful when engaging with others.
- Practice gratitude (see Chapter 11).

Relaxation Techniques

It is good to try and introduce some kind of relaxation into your daily schedule. There are also a number of specific relaxation exercises you can try, described next. You can try out some of these techniques and see what feels best for you. Relaxation is a skill that needs to be learned and practiced, so try not to worry about how well you are doing it or if it is working. These techniques are most effective if you can practice them regularly when you are in a calm state. It is almost like building a new muscle; the more you practice them, the more useful they will become, and the quicker they will kick in when you are feeling stressed.

General Tips for Relaxation Exercises

- Plan for some specific time to do your relaxation exercise.
- Prioritize this time as you would a work commitment.

- If you only have 5 minutes, that's okay; it can still be very useful.
- Find somewhere quiet and peaceful where you won't be disturbed.
- Sit or lie down somewhere comfortable.

Controlled Breathing

You may have noticed that when we are stressed our breath becomes more shallow and rapid. It is not uncommon to feel "air hunger" along with an inability to get a deep enough breath during times of stress and emotional exhaustion. Normal "unconscious" breathing typically involves the diaphragm and results in the rise and fall of your abdomen with each breath, but during stressful situations we may consciously begin using our chest muscles to breathe. This can result in unsatisfying breaths, and ultimately can lead to chest tightness and pain as a result of overusing the accessory muscles of your chest. Controlled breathing exercises can help return you to normal breathing and have demonstrated benefits for people with health-related breathing problems.[9] By slowing your breathing down you can reset the *alarm system* in the body. In turn, this will slow the heart rate and send the message to the brain that you are safe after all. Try this technique as soon as you start to feel overwhelmed or anxious. You can also practice it daily to reduce your baseline anxiety levels.

Place one hand on your stomach and the other on your chest. Try to breathe so that you can feel the air reaching all the way down to your stomach. It can help to imagine that you are inflating a balloon in your stomach. Be sure to feel your abdomen rise with your inhale and fall with your exhale.

Breathing Exercise

Step 1—Breathe out.
Step 2—Breathe in slowly for four counts.
Step 3—Hold your breath for four counts (or for however many feel comfortable for you).
Step 4—Breathe out slowly.
Repeat for several minutes.

Full-Body Relaxation: Jacobson's[10] Progressive Muscle Relaxation

When we feel stressed, we often carry tension in our muscles. Progressive muscular relaxation[11] is an evidence-based relaxation technique that has been found to reduce symptoms of anxiety and depression in cardiac patients. It makes you aware of that tension so you can let it go. Practice this exercise regularly to make it easier to let go of any tension.

Full-Body Relaxation Exercise

- Sit or lie down and make yourself comfortable.
- Breathe in, clench your right hand, and notice the tension in your hand. Breathe out and relax your hand, noticing the difference.
- Breathe in, clench your left hand, and notice the tension. Breathe out, relax, and notice the difference. Notice how comfortably heavy your hands and arms feel when you let them relax.
- Breathe in and "shrug" your shoulders to your ears; notice the tension in your shoulders and neck. Breathe out, relax, and notice the difference.
- Breathe in and tense your jaw; notice the tension in your mouth and jaw. Breathe out and notice how comfortable your whole face feels as you allow it to relax.
- Breathe in and lift your eyebrows, wrinkling your forehead; notice the tension. Breathe out, relax, and notice the difference.
- Breathe in and squeeze your eyes closed; notice the tension around your eyes. Breathe out, relax, and notice the difference.
- Breathe in and push your shoulders back; notice the tension. Breathe out, relax, and notice the difference.
- Breathe in, clench your stomach muscles, and notice the tension. Breathe out, relax, and notice the difference.
- Breathe in, bend your feet up, and notice the tension in your legs and feet. Breathe out, relax, and notice the difference.
- Breathe in and point your toes; notice the tension in your legs and feet. Breathe out, relax, and notice the difference. Allow the relaxation to deepen. Notice the pleasurable sensation of heaviness in your legs and arms as you relax them.
- Continue to relax, breathing calmly, using deep breathing.

Mindfulness and Meditation

Mindfulness has been found to benefit people living with chronic illness by reducing symptoms of anxiety, depression, and pain while improving overall well-being.[12] When we feel anxious, usually our minds are focused on something that has happened in the past, or we are preoccupied by concerns about something that is going to happen in the future. Mindfulness can help by training our minds to stay in the present moment or *being mode*. This is useful for managing anxiety, including generalized anxiety, social and health anxiety, obsessive compulsive disorder (OCD), or during a panic attack. Practicing mindfulness daily can also help to keep your baseline anxiety levels down.

Mindfulness techniques involve focusing on our five senses—sights, sounds, tastes, smells, and touch—to help us focus on the present moment. We encourage you to do this nonjudgmentally, accepting that while our minds will wander we can gently bring them back to the present moment each time this happens. While the practice of mindfulness may seem simple, it does take a lot of practice because it is so different from how our minds usually work.[13]

There are a wide variety of mindfulness practices that you can try. Next you will find a simple Mindfulness Breathing Exercise and Mindfulness Activity to try.

Mindfulness Breathing Exercise

Make sure you are sitting or lying comfortably and bring your attention to your breath, placing one hand on your stomach. Imagine there is a balloon in your stomach that inflates each time you breathe in. Notice the sensations in your body as you breathe in and out. Thoughts will come to your mind, and that is okay. Try to just notice them without judgment and pull your attention back to your breath. Repeat this process, breathing in and out. You can build up the time you spend on this exercise.

Mindfulness Activity

Choose a normal daily activity; this might be making a cup of tea, eating an apple, going for a walk, or lying in your bed drifting off to sleep. The next time you do this try to keep yourself in the present moment. Pay close attention to what you are doing. What do you smell? See? Hear? Taste? What do you feel? Again, thoughts will enter your mind but just notice them nonjudgmentally, let them go, and shift your attention back to what you are doing. Stay in the present moment and fully experience it, just being in the here and now.

Meditation

Meditation is a simple practice available to everyone; it's an act, generally practiced regularly, which can help us to develop the ability to become more calm and mindful in our day-to-day life. Regular meditation practice is said to have mental and physical health benefits. There are many different types of meditation techniques which are influenced by a variety of traditions, cultures, religions, and spiritual beliefs. Meditation doesn't need to be complicated or time consuming, and you don't need special clothes or training. Many begin with practice slowly at first for 5 minutes or so, and then may choose to build up the time slowly. The goal isn't to empty your mind completely, but rather to release any crowded thoughts you may have that may be causing stress. As with any type of activity, be sure to speak with your healthcare provider about the possible risks and benefits in relation to your health situation. Some examples of ways to meditate:

• Daily walks in nature
• Daily prayer
• Reading poetry or scripture and reflecting
• Guided meditation in a class or on an app
• Yoga
• Qi gong
• Tai chi
• Deep, calm breathing

Distraction

Distraction helps by taking our attention away from our distressing feelings, for example when you are sitting in a doctor's waiting area or when you feel overwhelmed with worrying thoughts. Distraction has been shown to help to reduce anxiety levels and distress, for example during conscious medical procedures.[14] By distracting yourself you can keep distress levels in check and help to prevent a panic attack or cycle of anxiety (e.g., health anxiety or OCD). Distraction is not the same as suppressing your feelings. You are still validating any normal emotional response to the situation. However, you are shifting the focus of your attention to something less distressing. Different things work for different people and we have listed some suggestions next.

Distraction Techniques

- Doing a puzzle (e.g., crossword, word search, sudoku)
- Coloring or practicing a form of art
- Calling or messaging someone for a chat
- Reading a magazine
- Watching TV
- Listening to music
- Going for a walk
- Spending time with your pet
- Counting backward from 50 to 0, 100 to 0
- Doing the alphabet backward

Keep It in Check: Worry Time

Some people who experience a lot of worrying thoughts, especially about their health, find it helps to set aside a certain time or times each day, for about 10–15 minutes, to simply "worry."[15] During this time it can be helpful to keep a journal to jot down whatever is concerning you. We recommend also using that time to separate the worries into two columns: what you can control and what you cannot control (see worry tree, Figure 5.1).[16]

If you feel up to continuing the process, the next step would be to make a plan for taking care of the things you can control. For the list of those you cannot control, meditation and emotional release can help you to let them go. When worries pop up at other times of the day or night, you can remind yourself that you will come back to them and make a plan to deal with them later during your scheduled worry time. You don't need to get into an "argument" with yourself; rather, try to mindfully notice the worry,

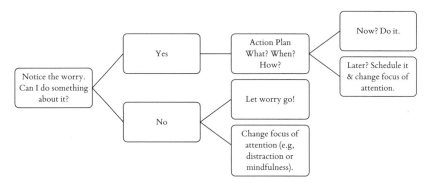

Figure 5.1 Worry tree (Butler and Hope 1995).[17]

like a little cloud floating by, and gently shift your focus of attention back to what you are doing or something distracting. Initially this can be difficult, but with practice it becomes easier. This strategy helps to contain the worrying thoughts at a set time each day rather than allowing them to take over your life.

6

Managing Uncomfortable Feelings

Between stimulus and response there is a space. In that space is our power to choose our response. In our response lies our growth and our freedom.

—Viktor Frankl[1]

Research suggests that fostering healthy emotional regulation can help to prevent mental health problems. Emotional regulation is the ability to effectively monitor, evaluate, and modify our emotions, which is fundamental to everyday functioning. This includes having an awareness of and being able to identify our emotions, being able to tolerate unpleasant feelings, recognize patterns, and having the ability to manage them in a healthy way. Emotional regulation isn't something we are born with. It is a set of skills that we can build on to improve our emotional intelligence (EQ), health, and well-being.[2]

Our emotions tell us important information. For example, we feel sad when we experience loss, and we feel angry when we feel that something unfair has happened (see Table 6.1). It is helpful to listen to our bodies and what messages our feelings are telling us. When we are able to do that proactively (instead of reactively), we can respond to the situation in a thoughtful and empathetic way. It is possible to build on your emotional regulation skills using the techniques in this chapter.

Table 6.1 Emotional Messages: What Our Feelings Are Trying to Tell Us

Emotion	Physical Symptoms	Message
Sad	De-energized, thinking the worst, heavy, numb, tired	I have lost something important to me; I can't deal with this. (e.g., in response to news that your health condition has deteriorated)
Anxious	Racing thoughts, sweating, racing heart; fight, flight, or freeze	I am in danger; something bad is going to happen. (e.g., ahead of an invasive or surgical procedure or hospital appointment)
Angry	Racing thoughts, tense muscles, heart racing, rapid breathing; fight, flight, or freeze	Something unfair has happened to me. (e.g., finding out a medical intervention is needed or missing out on something because of your health)
Guilty	Self-critical thoughts, sweating, racing heart; fight, flight, or freeze	I've done something wrong. (e.g., "I wish I would have taken better care of myself!")
Joyful	Energized and hopeful	I like this, it is important to me, life is good. (e.g., being discharged from the hospital and feeling joyful about going home and getting on with life)
Contentment	Present focused, calm, relaxed	I am peaceful and satisfied. (e.g., feeling like you are managing your condition and getting the most out of life)

Accepting Uncertainty and Normalizing Distress

It turns out that our emotions have a helpful role to play. They are our body's way of giving us important messages. Often we try to suppress or resist distressing emotions. This is understandable; however, psychology research suggests that when we try to suppress how we are feeling, it can actually make the feeling more intense. This can lead to unhealthy coping strategies such as binge eating, drinking too much, or risk-taking behaviors. When we ignore them, often the feelings intensify to try and make us listen. By learning to accept normal emotional responses to difficult life experiences, sometimes termed "radical acceptance,"[3] we can validate our feelings, learn to manage them, and problem-solve what we need to do to feel better.[4]

For example, feelings of vulnerability and anxiety are a normal response to feeling unsafe, under threat, and uncertain. It is actually normal and okay to feel anxious when you face uncertainty. Often we find this difficult to accept and seek reassurance from others, by searching for answers or engaging in checking behaviors such as looking for bodily symptoms. However, this only provides a quick fix and makes us focus even more on our anxious feelings. Learning to accept that life is full of uncertainty, especially for those of us with a congenital heart condition (CHC), is an important skill.

> *Throughout my entire life I was told by my doctors that I was one of their oldest patients with my type of CHC. They weren't able to answer many of my questions about my long-term prognosis. At first that was really scary for me. At some point I learned to embrace the uncertainty, and it became my friend. I learned to balance the not knowing with some hope. No one really knows what the future holds; who knows, I could surprise them all.*
>
> —Alex, 54 years old, United States

Labeling Your Emotions

Rather than suppressing or resisting your feelings, research has shown that exploring and labeling our emotions helps to make them less distressing.[5] It is important to learn how to recognize your emotions and label them because they carry important messages about what you need. First, ask yourself, "What is this feeling and where am I experiencing it in my body?" If you are having difficulty naming the emotion you are experiencing, we suggest that you try to use an emotion wheel, or wheel of emotions, which is a visual tool to help individuals identify and verbalize their emotions. It is also a way to understand the relationship and intensity of different emotions. There are a number of versions of this wheel on the Internet.

Instead of pushing away distressing feelings, you can say to yourself, "I don't want this feeling, but I can stand it" and rather than fighting it, just let it come and go, accepting it. Emotions, similar to clouds in the sky, will eventually pass. You just have to find something to help you wait it out. While you are doing that we suggest finding a way to tolerate the discomfort. Some people do this by physical exercise, walking, taking a warm bath, talking to someone supportive, or journaling.

Once the feeling is named, the next step is to identify what has triggered it. Sometimes that means really meditating on it and peeling back the layers. Ask yourself, "When did this feeling begin? What triggered it? Why am I feeling this way?" This is how we learn from our feelings. Your feelings then become an ally, telling you what you need, rather than your enemy.

This process sometimes takes a little while; it is a layered approach to processing your emotions. Doing this can put you in a better position to understand what your body is telling you and then makes it easier for you to make a plan for feeling better. By recognizing your feelings, you can also find healthy ways to express them rather than being controlled by them. It is useful to evaluate whether the trigger is something you can control or something you cannot control. If you can control it, then the best next step may be to make a plan for change. If it is something you cannot control, then some of the techniques we've provided here will help you let it go. The following sentence can help you better link your feelings, their triggers, and what you can do to help yourself.

I feel ... because ... and I need ...

For example, I feel *scared* because *I am going back to the hospital for a checkup*, and I need *to take someone supportive with me*.

Know Your Triggers

One way to significantly cut down on stressful situations and feelings is to get to know your triggers. A trigger is a situation that may provoke a bad memory, or uncomfortable feelings and unhelpful behaviors. Once these situations are identified, it will be easier for you to take steps to either minimize your exposure to them and/or prepare yourself to manage the feelings they evoke. If you are unsure, it can help to keep a diary detailing what you are doing, where you are, who you are with, and what thoughts are going through your mind when you start to feel distressed. Over time you may start to notice patterns about what your triggers are and that can help you make sense of what is going on for you. That will enable you to put strategies in place to manage your difficult feelings during those times.

Sarah noticed that she was eating more junk food, getting easily irritated by her family, and had withdrawn from her friends. She took some time to reflect and recognized she had been feeling low, irritable, and tense since receiving an appointment letter for an annual cardiology check a week ago. She realized that she was feeling nervous about the appointment. Instead of bottling her feelings up like she usually did, she went online to discuss them in a CHC chat group. She also explained her worries to her partner, who offered to take a day off work and accompany her to the appointment. Through this process she decided to focus more on self-care to manage her understandable increase in stress levels.

Managing Your Emotions

Emotional release is finding a healthy way to express how you are feeling. This might be writing it down, punching a pillow, or "getting it off your chest" by talking to a trusted friend. Other strategies include exercise such as going for a fast walk, playing a musical instrument, or using art as a way of expressing yourself. Finding healthy ways to communicate how you are feeling, such as speaking assertively to others (see Chapter 8), is also essential. Having a good cry is another great way to release your emotions. Crying is a way to release the stress hormone cortisol, and it may activate our parasympathetic nervous system, which helps our body to rest and feel calmer.

Managing Overwhelming Emotions

The techniques described next can help to reduce the intensity of distressing feelings. It can be helpful to pair these techniques with the Controlled Breathing Exercise, described earlier in Chapter 5.

Live One Day at a Time

If you are having a lot of anxiety and worry about the worst scenario, try to stay in the moment and not think more than one day or even one hour at a time. Sometimes thinking too far into the future can really increase uncomfortable feelings.

Positive Affirmations, Coping Statements, and Self-Compassion

Self-compassion is increasingly being linked to good mental health.[6] Positive coping statements can help us get through distressing emotions.

Some statements that may help are listed here. It could be helpful to add some of your own by asking yourself what you would like someone to say to you when you feel distressed and write down the answer. If that is too difficult to do, ask yourself what you would say to a friend or child in a similar situation. Here are some examples of the affirmations that have been helpful to some and that you can draw on the next time you feel this way.

- This will pass.
- Feelings are normal and temporary.
- My feelings are valid.
- I got through this before.
- This feels bad, but it is a normal human response, and it will pass.
- Everything is temporary.
- I am allowed to feel upset.
- I am a good and worthwhile person.
- My life has meaning and purpose.
- I can deal with this.
- I am good enough.
- This is tough; what do I need to do to cope or feel better?
- I am worthy.
- I am more than my accomplishments or failures.
- It is okay to cry.
- Everyone makes mistakes.
- Even though I am feeling this, I accept myself.

It can be hard to remember these statements when you are feeling overwhelmed. It might help to write some of them on a card and keep it somewhere safe, such as your wallet or phone, to look at the next time you are feeling distressed. You might also want to hang some inspirational affirmations around your home as reminders.

Grounding Exercises

Sometimes when Kirsty goes to the hospital, the smells and sounds take her right back to recovering from heart surgery on the childrens' ward and she feels overwhelmed. She tries to take a moment to slow her breathing and ground herself in the here and now. She carries a stone in her pocket as a "grounding object" that she holds onto as she repeats coping statements reminding herself that as an adult she has more control, that she has coped before, that it is okay and understandable to feel anxious, and that she will be back home soon.

Grounding exercises are a way to bring yourself back to the present moment when you become overwhelmed by distressing feelings. They are especially useful for people who are experiencing intense emotions or are recovering from traumatic experiences. Grounding exercises can help if you are feeling very anxious, for example during a panic attack or if you go into the "freeze" response. They are also useful if you are feeling angry, upset, or frightened or when you experience a flashback, nightmare, intrusive memory, or ruminating thoughts. Grounding can be used anywhere at any time and no one else needs to know you are doing it.

5, 4, 3, 2, 1 Method

Describe (out loud if possible) five things you can see, four things you can touch, three things you can hear, two things you can smell, and one thing you can taste.

Grounding Object

A grounding object is a comforting item that carries a positive meaning for you that you can use to distract yourself if you feel overwhelmed by focusing on the color and textures of the object. It should be small enough to carry with you, such as a pebble, soft piece of cloth, or necklace.

Grounding Phrase

You can also come up with a phrase to remind you that you are living in the present moment. This might be something like *I have survived the past, and I am safe now* or *I am strong and have faith that I will get through this.* It is important to come up with a phrase that is meaningful for you. It can be useful to write it down and keep it somewhere so you can look at it when you feel overwhelmed.

Grounding Activities

Other ways to ground yourself in the present include running cool water over your hands and noticing how it feels, reaching out to touch objects around you, noticing your body and how it feels while sitting or standing. Make use of aromatherapy by using essential oils or a diffuser. You can also think about your own strategies to ground yourself in the present moment.

Somatic Exercises

Clearing a Space[7]

- Lie down or sit in a way that's comfortable for you and loosen any clothing that is too tight.
- Pay attention to your breathing (try the breathing exercise described previously for a few minutes).
- Ask yourself, "What's between me and feeling perfectly all right?"
- Spend a moment with this issue, noticing how you carry it in your body for a few seconds.
- Think about how this issue physically manifests as a tension in your body.
- Ask yourself, "What is the 'feel' of this thing?"
- Don't try to go into the issue or try to solve the problem; just notice how it feels in your body.
- Try to find some words or an image for the feeling or the "quality," for example "scared, frustrating, annoying."
- Imagine wrapping this issue—the physical tension, and the feelings it brings up—like a parcel and set it outside of yourself for a moment.
- You may experience a "sigh" of relief as you imagine lifting it and setting it outside.
- See if you can set it outside for a while.
- You can come back and solve it later, but for now see if your body can be free of it for a moment.
- Repeat this process for any other items that you are carrying.
- Continue in this way until all the issues have been named and set outside yourself.
- Enjoy the experience of the "cleared space" in your body.
- You may want to create a word or an image for this good feeling state, so that you can come back here whenever you want.

The Diver's Response

When mammals hit the cold water, it automatically triggers a physiological relaxation response. It is especially effective and useful when in an extreme emotional state. Before you try this we recommend getting the okay from your cardiologist as this simple technique will bring down your adrenaline, calm your breathing, and slow your heart rate. One way to initiate this is by taking a cold shower and making sure to get the cold water on your face. A quicker way to get this response is to grab something cold like a soft drink can or a cold wet cloth and place it on or over your face.

Pelvic Floor Exercise

One of our body's secret weapons is our vagus nerve,[8] one of the cranial nerves which connects the brain to the body. Some techniques can trigger the vagal brake, which slows down the fight or flight system, leading to a relaxation response. One way to obtain this response is by relaxing your pelvic floor muscles. Before you try this exercise we recommend that you empty your bladder. Otherwise, it may feel uncomfortable.

1. Sit comfortably, either with your eyes open or closed.
2. Imagine your pelvic bones, your tail bone, the space between them— that is your pelvic floor.
3. Begin breathing deeply and comfortably.
4. Begin to completely let go of all tension in your pelvic area (opposite of Kegel exercises).
5. Focus on relaxing your pelvic area, which will release the tension around your vagus nerve.
6. Do this for 1–3 minutes.

Sighing

We naturally sigh or yawn a few times each hour. Sighing can help to rest the autonomic nervous system. You can induce the exaggerated inhale and exhale of a sigh or yawn.

Stretching

Stretching is such an underrated stress reliever. You may have noticed stretching and yawning are actions that pets use a lot to relieve stress (how often have you seen your dog or cat stretching it out?). It automatically releases muscle tension and can help with body aches. There is no prescribed routine or time requirement, and there are many different stretches you can find online, depending upon the body parts that need attention.

Increasing Feelings of Psychological Safety

If you want to change the world, start by making people feel safer.

—Stephen Porges

Feeling safe is important for psychological health and well-being.[9] Soothing techniques draw on the senses to make you feel safer. They can be different for each of us. You can enhance feelings of safety by holding in mind comforting images, looking at photographs from a happy and relaxing time, thinking about someone who offered you unconditional love and acceptance, going for a walk in nature, watching something comforting on TV, feeling something soothing such as a cozy or weighted blanket or comfortable clothing, or holding a grounding object such as a pebble or stroking a pet. Smells can also be soothing, such as using a relaxing moisturizer, candle, or essential oils; enjoying the scents of nature; or noticing the aroma of something baking. Comforting sounds may also help, such as birdsong, relaxing music, or your own favorites.

> *The last time Laura went into hospital to have her pacemaker replaced she took a kit of items that she knew would help her. This included photos of her family, relaxing aromatherapy spray, moisturizer, comfortable pajamas, puzzle books, magazines, snacks, and some card games she could play with my family and young kids when they visited.*

You can create a soothing box where you keep all of the things that help you feel safer; you can turn to this box when you are feeling overwhelmed. You may find it helpful to create a bag of soothing items like this to take with you during a hospital stay.

Safe Place—Guided Visualization

Guided visualization has been shown to reduce levels of anxiety, for example before surgery.[10] It can help to create a safe place in your mind. This can be based on a real experience, or it can be imagined. It is a place where you feel happy and secure. For example, it might be lying on a beach or in front of a cozy fire. Use all your senses to make this as real as possible. Think about the colors, skin sensations, what you can touch, what you can smell, what you can hear. For example, imagine a gentle breeze, the feeling of the sun on your skin, the sound of the waves lapping. You may find it helpful to take some time to describe your safe place in as much detail as possible, drawing on all of your senses. Sometimes writing a description of your safe place helps in this process. There are lots of free ways to access guided visualization exercises online or on meditation apps.

Managing Anger

Sometimes we don't recognize we are carrying anger around with us. We may hear feedback from family or friends to let us know that we seem more irritable than usual or find that we are less tolerant and generally more frustrated. If this is something you can relate to, then perhaps unexpressed anger could be the cause.

The first step in dealing with anger is recognizing it. The next step is uncovering the trigger. Anger is a normal response to a sense of injustice or feeling like something unfair has happened. There are various challenges that may legitimately trigger this feeling as a result of living with a CHC or that may have been triggered by something else entirely. Figuring out the source of your anger can often help you in the process of releasing it. Undiagnosed neurocognitive issues such as attention-deficit/hyperactivity disorder (ADHD), dyslexia, or dyspraxia can contribute to daily frustrations that can trigger angry outbursts. Since neurocognitive difficulties are more common in people with a CHC, it might be useful to ask your healthcare providers to refer you for a neurocognitive assessment for this to be ruled out if you find daily tasks leave you feeling frustrated.

Tips for Managing Anger

- Be thoughtful of the words and the tone that you use.
- Increase your awareness of the first physical signs of anger (tight jaw, raised shoulders).
- Try to express yourself when you are calm and well rested, and make sure you aren't hungry (or hangry). This will set you up for a productive conversation with the recipient; draw on the section on assertive communication styles in Chapter 8.

- Do some deep breathing or use a mantra such as "Breathe in calm, breathe out anger" if your temper is flaring up.
- Use "I" statements. This will help you avoid using blame and criticism. Take a time-out if you need a few minutes to compose yourself; step away from the situation and count to 10 (or 100!).
- Journaling or letter writing is a great alternative for when you aren't comfortable talking about it, or if you are processing a past trauma as the cause.
- Use humor to release any tension.
- Get physical. Go for a walk or do some stretching.

Therapeutic Letter Writing

Sometimes we project our feelings of frustration and hurt about one thing onto something or someone else. Often this is because we have not had the opportunity to safely express our feelings when they were triggered or because we were silenced or invalidated when we tried to. Or it may be because the person we want to talk to is no longer with us due to bereavement. Identifying the real trigger for your feelings of anger, hurt, sadness, fear, or frustration and finding a safe way to process your feelings can help you to let them go without damaging other relationships and opportunities in the here and now. Writing a letter (one that you won't actually send) can be a powerful means to this end, providing an opportunity to make sense of bottled-up feelings.

Therapeutic Letter-Writing Exercise

- Find a safe time and space where you won't be interrupted.
- Get a pen and paper or a computer and write a letter to the person or people who triggered your feelings (e.g., a workplace or childhood bully, a medical professional who wouldn't listen, a critical parent, or even the universe for the cards you've been dealt).
- Be as expressive as you can; don't worry about making sense, jumping about through different timelines, spelling, or grammar. The purpose is to have the opportunity to find your voice, tell your side of the story, and express your feelings.

- Write down how you were made to feel (at the time and now) and the impact this event(s) has had on you.
- This can be a very emotive task, so you may want to do it in short chunks (5–10 minutes), putting the letter away and coming back to it when you feel ready.
- You may also find that, as you process one thing, other events come to mind; you want to add these because often difficult emotions are layered.
- As you are processing your feelings, you may feel more emotional and dream and think about the event(s) more than usual. This is okay; it means you are processing what has happened. Be self-compassionate, look after yourself, and draw from the techniques in this book about safe emotional release.
- When you feel the letter is finished, add a final paragraph stating that you will no longer be consumed by what happened, that you are moving forward positively, and taking control of your life on your terms. It doesn't matter if you don't feel like this yet; this is your first step toward liberating yourself from these past hurts.
- If there is someone in your life whom you can trust, such as a partner, parent, or therapist, you may want to share the letter with them. Having someone bear witness to your story can be therapeutic; however, this step is not necessary for positive change.
- You may instead choose to do something symbolic, such as burning the letter, to mark moving forward and letting go.

7

Managing Unhelpful Thoughts and Behaviors

Coping can be messy, and that is okay. Generally speaking, we are not always aware of the impact that our thoughts, feelings, and behaviors have (see Figure 7.1). Yet our thoughts have a big impact on how we interpret and feel about the things that happen to us and how we respond to them. Most of the time we take for granted that the conscious thoughts going through our mind are "facts" and the feelings they evoke inform what we should do about them. We may go on "autopilot," responding in the same way that we have always done without reflecting on whether this is really the best or only option.

Generally, we can't waste time and energy having to analyze everything that happens to us. Sometimes we fall into unhelpful patterns of thinking and behaviors that hold us back in life or no longer serve our needs. Unhelpful beliefs, about ourselves, other people, or the world, may underlie these thoughts and contribute to health anxiety, panic, low mood, or other mental health problems. We may then develop ways of managing distress that seem like a quick fix but end up creating their own problems. We may have learned these responses when we were young children and had fewer options, but they may no longer be the best option available to us. These strategies might have become habitual, even problematic, maintaining our psychological distress.

For example, worry-checking behaviors and reassurance seeking, such as continually checking your pulse, can create an illusion of certainty and sense of control but can get out of hand. We may use strategies to block out difficult feelings such as risk taking, drinking too much alcohol, smoking or vaping, overeating or undereating, and misusing prescribed or nonprescribed drugs. If we feel overwhelmed or poorly understood, we might

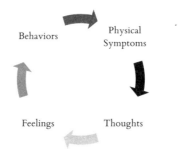

Figure 7.1 Cycle of behaviors, thoughts, feelings and physical symptoms.

withdraw from social contact, but this can give us more time to ruminate and consolidate feelings of isolation which can lead to low mood. In this chapter we will consider the link between thoughts, feelings, and behaviors, how we can end up stuck in a vicious cycle of distress, and how to break the cycle.

The Interaction between Our Thoughts, Feelings, and Behaviors

Andrea struggled to keep up with her friends at school and grew up feeling like she was an "outsider." To fit in, she tried to please everyone. As an adult, she still tried really hard to keep everyone happy but felt anxious if anyone was critical or seemed displeased with her. For a few days, after this happened she would feel low and un-motivated. She would cancel plans, withdraw socially, and miss out on enjoyable ex-periences. It impacted her physically, too, and she felt lethargic and found herself comfort eating. Over time, because she was doing less and less, this seemed to confirm her original thought that she was an "outsider" and she slipped into a deep depression.

This is known as a vicious cycle of depression. It is possible to break these cycles by challenging unhelpful negative thoughts and behaviors, detailed in the following sections.

Address Unhelpful Thinking Styles

Unhelpful thinking styles (cognitive distortions) often keep us feeling low or anxious and can result in a "negative downward spiral."[1] Over time they can become a habit keeping us stuck in a negative cycle. We have listed common unhelpful thinking styles in Table 7.1. It can help to identify them and rather than accepting these thoughts as facts to start to recognize and challenge them to develop a more realistic perspective (cognitive correction).

Table 7.1 Common Cognitive Distortions

Cognitive Distortion	Description	Example
Personalizing	The belief that negative things others do or say are in direct or indirect response to you.	*Someone is offhand, and you assume they don't like you.*
Mental filter	Noticing only what fits with your negative bias and ignoring anything positive or anything that challenges it.	*Focusing on the one mistake you made and dismissing everything that went well.*
Jumping to conclusions	Believing you know how others feel about you, or you can predict how someone will act or how an outcome will turn out, also called "fortune telling."	*Assuming that you will fail a class, so "why bother" signing up.*
Catastrophizing	Assuming the worst possible outcome.	*Being 5 minutes late for work and assuming you will be sacked.*
Black-and-white thinking	Only seeing things as extremes, or as "all or nothing" with no shades in between.	*"If I am not a perfect student, I am a failure."*
Shoulds and musts	These appear as rules to live by which cannot be changed; this can be directed at yourself or at others.	*"I should cook dinner every night" or "I shouldn't be so lazy."*
Overgeneralizing	Making a conclusion based on one negative event.	*You fail an exam and believe you are a terrible student and should drop out of school.*
Emotional reasoning	When your emotions take over and you believe that because you feel a certain way it must be true.	*Assuming because you feel anxious something bad will happen.*
Blaming	When you hold another person or situation responsible for any pain and life dissatisfaction, or they blame you for every problem that is out of their control.	*"It's my ex-boyfriend's fault that my life is not what I want it to be."*
Compare and despair	Comparing the worst of your life with the best of someone else's.	*Scrolling through social media and assuming everyone else has a perfect life.*

Common Cognitive Distortions

Challenging Unhelpful Thoughts: ABCDE

It is possible to challenge unhelpful thought patterns using the following technique.[2]

Attention—notice any unhelpful, negative thoughts.

Believe—don't just accept them as fact, but question whether you actually believe the thought.

Challenge—challenge the thought; the following questions might help:

- Consider the evidence for and against the thought to gain a more realistic perspective (it may help to write this down in two columns).
- Could there possibly be another alternative?
- What would a friend say about this thought?
- What would you say to a friend or loved one who was experiencing this thought?
- Will this matter in a week, a month, or a year's time?
- What is the worst that could happen, and how likely is that?
- Are you underestimating how well you would cope even if the worst did happen?
- What is the best that could happen?
- What is a more realistic perspective?
- How useful is this thought to you?

Discount—discount the thought if it is unrealistic, unhelpful, and lacks evidence. You may find it useful to use mindfulness techniques to observe the thought and "let it go" rather than getting stuck in a fight with it, thereby feeding it by giving it more attention.

Explore—carefully consider your options; don't just act out of habit (see section on "Addressing Unhelpful Behaviors").

Core Beliefs and Rules for Living

Often underlying the unhelpful thoughts described earlier are unfounded beliefs that we have formed about ourselves, other people, and the world, and the rules and strategies that we have developed to compensate for them.[3]

As children, we learn about ourselves based on our experiences and the messages we pick up; for example, "I have green eyes" or "I live in America." Mostly, these beliefs are accurate and harmless. However, sometimes, while perfectly understandable in light of our experiences, they are unhelpful and negative. For example, "I am unlovable," "I am different," or "I am a failure." It is important to note that these beliefs are not facts; they have often been formed through a child's eyes and sometimes come from an outside source (a toxic relative, peers, or social expectations in the media). As social animals, often these beliefs and rules reflect what we needed to do as children to feel loved or accepted, or they were just ingrained in us if we were exposed to that type of messaging (such as "boys don't cry" or "being assertive isn't ladylike"). As adults, it is likely that some of these internal thoughts are holding us back and contributing to low self-esteem, anxiety, and low mood. As a rule of thumb, if you feel like your emotional response to a situation is disproportionate, then it is likely one of these unhelpful beliefs has been triggered.

To compensate for these unhelpful beliefs, we may form "rules" such as "I won't reveal my true self or I will be rejected" or "I can't make any mistakes or I will get caught out." While these rules may have seemed to help us out at one time, it is likely that they are outdated, keep the original negative belief in place, and hold you back in life. Further, they may contribute to unhelpful "compensatory" behaviors, keeping you stuck in a vicious cycle.

Sam struggled throughout school due to undiagnosed dyslexia and attention-deficit/hyperactivity disorder (ADHD). He was always getting into trouble and falling behind his classmates. He fundamentally felt like he was a failure, and as an adult he over-compensated by trying to avoid making mistakes. Sam set up his own business as an electrician working hard and on the surface appeared to be successful. However, he didn't allow himself to show any vulnerability and drove himself to exhaustion with "perfectionist" behaviors and self-criticism. His apparent drive was fueled with anxiety about making any mistakes. As such, he never challenged the underlying unhelpful belief that he was a failure and he felt like an imposter. No matter what he achieved he just kept setting the bar higher for himself, waiting to be "found out." Eventually, he pushed himself to exhaustion and started to experience panic attacks. Only then did he reach out to a therapist, who helped him to recognize that he had never been a failure, providing the opportunity for him to challenge his relentless high standards and liberate himself to live life more freely and make human errors just like everyone else. He was then in a position to get a diagnosis for ADHD and dyslexia, and this enabled him to make sense of his experiences, access support, and develop useful coping strategies.

Table 7.2 Unhelpful Beliefs

Unhelpful Belief	Unhelpful Rules (Examples)
I am unlovable.	I must hide my true self, or I will be rejected.
I am different.	I must not share my own needs, or I will be rejected.
I am a failure.	I must never make any mistakes, or I will be found out.
I am stupid.	I must keep my opinions to myself, or I will be found out.
I am fragile.	I must be very careful at all times, or I won't be able to cope.
I am a burden.	I must suppress my own needs and keep everyone else happy, or I won't be loved.

Common Unhelpful Beliefs and Rules for Living

By recognizing unhelpful core beliefs and the rules we follow to compensate for them we can start to challenge them (see Table 7.2). This takes time because it involves relearning the habits of a lifetime. The following steps can help (also see Table 7.3).

Tips for Challenging Core Belief and Rules

- Write out what you think your unhelpful beliefs and rules might be. Beliefs usually are "I am . . ." statements, while rules are often "I should / must . . . or else . . ." statements (we have listed some common ones here, which may help).
- Score them out and replace them with what you would prefer them to be (go for a more realistic alternative; you don't need to believe it just now).
- If you are struggling with this, think about what you would say to a child, friend, or loved one.
- Keep your new belief and rule somewhere that you can see them and repeat them to yourself.
- Start "acting" as if your new beliefs and behavior are true (fake it till you make it!).
- It might help to set yourself small challenges to test your new rule (e.g., purposefully leave a mess, open up about your feelings more than usual, be more assertive).
- Don't give yourself a hard time for falling into old habits; this will take time.

Table 7.3 Alternatives to Unhelpful Beliefs and Rules

Unhelpful Belief and Alternative	Unhelpful Rule and Alternative
I am unlovable.	*I must hide my true self, or I will be rejected.*
I am lovable.	I can be my true self; people who care about me will still want me.
I am different.	*I must not share my own needs, or I will be rejected.*
I am no more different than anyone else.	I can share my needs; people who matter will still want me.
I am a failure.	*I must never make any mistakes, or I will be found out.*
I am good enough.	Everyone makes mistakes; as long as I try my best that is enough.
I am stupid.	*I must keep my opinions to myself, or I will be found out.*
I am trying my best, and that's all anyone can do.	Trying my best is good enough.

Health Beliefs

Understandably we may have developed beliefs and rules for living about our health in light of our congenital heart condition (CHC). While there is little doubt these beliefs and rules will make sense in terms of our (often childhood) experiences, they may be outdated or limiting us in the here and now (see Table 7.4).

> As a child, Jenny (45 years old) had been medically advised to abstain from gym lessons and active play. Consequently, she'd always felt "different" and "fragile" and worried about pushing her body in case she fell unwell and needed to go back to the hospital. Yet at her last routine cardiology appointment her cardiologist encouraged her to exercise. While she wanted to, she felt confused and anxious. She explained this was contrary to what she had been told growing up. Her cardiologist agreed to arrange an exercise stress test to help her understand her physical limits and referred her to a specialist physiotherapist to help her to develop an exercise plan that met her needs. By working with the physiotherapist she gradually built up her confidence in her body.

It is important to note that sometimes our unhelpful beliefs and rules are grounded in painful childhood experiences. This means they can be difficult to "let go" unless we have time to process the feelings they evoke. If this is the case it may be helpful to work through things with a qualified therapist.

Table 7.4 Unhelpful Health Beliefs

Unhelpful Health Belief	Alternative Belief
I can't trust my body.	My body has been through a lot; I can work with it.
There is no point listening to my body because it lets me down.	Learning to listen to and work with my body will help me manage my health and feel better.
I am defective.	I am normal; I just happen to have been born with a heart condition.
There are lots of things I can't do, and there is no point even trying.	I can work with my body and take care of myself to reach my full potential.
I don't deserve the same in life as "normal" people.	I matter just as much as everyone else.
I am a burden.	I have a lot to offer others.
I must suppress my own needs and keep everyone else happy or I won't be loved.	My needs are just as important as everyone else's.
My life has been so difficult; I have nothing to look forward to.	There is no reason to believe that my life can't improve.
I am fragile.	I have a health condition that I can manage.
I can't cope.	I can learn how to manage my condition and make the most of my life.

Myth Busting: Some Common Misconceptions about Congenital Heart Conditions

Often the worries, thoughts, and beliefs we have about our condition come from misconceptions about health and well-being in wider society. We have listed some common social myths that are untrue and can be harmful to us:

Myth—*People with a CHC often have life-threatening arrhythmias, especially during exercise.*
Fact—Sudden cardiac death is actually very rare; if this is something that concerns you, please speak to your adult congenital heart disease specialist.
Myth—*People are either healthy or unwell.*
Fact—Health is on a continuum; most people lie somewhere in between, and this can vary over time and even day to day.
Myth—*People with a CHC can't have biological children.*
Fact—Most people with a CHC can have biological children, but it is important this is planned under the guidance of specialist care. See Chapter 10.

Myth— *People with health conditions are a burden on society.*

Fact—Any one of us can be born with or develop a physical or psychological health condition. Many people live independently with their condition and contribute to society in many ways. Lived experience of adversity can also contribute to positive adaptation, making us more empathic and socially conscious.

Myth—*Why bother with (fill in the blank)? I won't be around long enough to enjoy the benefits.*

Fact—No one can predict the future. Work toward reaching your fullest potential, whether that involves education, employment, or committing to a relationship.

Myth—*There is no point looking after myself; my body has failed me.*

Fact—You are doing your best to overcome more challenges than most. Working with your body will enable you to feel your best and reach your fullest potential. Giving up will only make you feel worse.

Addressing Unhelpful Behaviors

Often we fall into patterns of behavior that seem like a quick fix but that end up keeping the problem going or even making it worse. For example, if we experience a panic attack, we may avoid returning to where it happened. This can get in the way of our day-to-day life, gradually chip away at our confidence, and leave us feeling like we can't cope. Over time we might start to avoid other places, too. Noticing and addressing these unhealthy behaviors early on puts us in a better position to regain control of our lives. Here we describe evidence-based strategies for addressing the most common unhelpful behaviors.

Evaluating Safety Behaviors

It is very common to cope with distressing feelings using safety behaviors. This is completely understandable; of course, we want to find safety when we feel uncomfortable. Commonly this involves either avoiding what is making you feel upset or seeking reassurance about it.[4] For example, someone who feels anxious around other people may avoid public places or only go to them with another person or at quiet times. Typical avoidance behaviors include canceling your plans, stopping doing things you used to, and going out of your way to avoid going somewhere or doing something that makes you feel uncomfortable (such as people, situations, or public speaking). Reassurance-seeking behaviors typically include ruminating about what you said or did, repeatedly asking others for feedback, making lots of lists, overpreparing, having an alcoholic drink or tranquilizer in an attempt to feel more relaxed, checking symptoms repeatedly, and looking things up on the Internet.

Unfortunately, over time, these quick-fix behaviors can undermine our confidence and make the distress or anxiety worse in the longer term. They can also get in the way of day-to-day life. For example, if you have a headache that you are worried about, Googling your symptoms seldom helps and can end up making you feel even more preoccupied by your concerns.

It is important to tackle these safety behaviors to rebuild your confidence. You can do this by developing an "exposure hierarchy" (see Figure 7.2). This involves making an end goal (e.g., going to the supermarket) and then developing a series of steps to get you there, starting from where you are now. For each step you can vary the *duration* (how long you will spend there), *who* you go with (such as your partner versus going alone), and *when* you go (when it is quiet versus when it is busy).

Exposure Hierarchy

Begin by stating your end goal and then break down how you will get there into achievable steps. Repeat each step until it no longer makes you feel anxious. Reward yourself every time you attempt a step and draw on techniques such as grounding, breathing exercises, and distraction to help to manage your anxiety. Don't worry if you go back a step or two; just try again.

You can gradually let go of reassurance-seeking and checking behaviors in a similar, step-by-step way. If you notice this is something that you do, you can try to hold off on doing it for a few minutes and distract yourself or use some grounding or breathing exercises. Often you find that once this time passes you no longer have the intense urge to ask for reassurance or carry out the checking behavior.

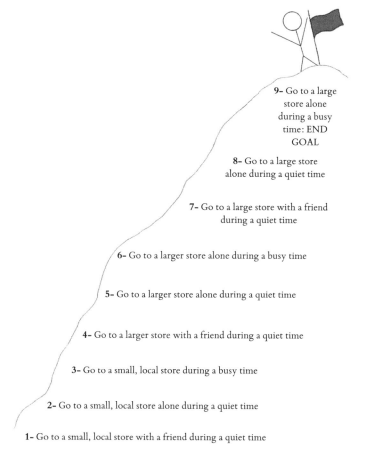

9- Go to a large
store alone
during a busy
time: END
GOAL

8- Go to a large store
alone during a quiet time

7- Go to a large store with a friend
during a quiet time

6- Go to a larger store alone during a busy time

5- Go to a larger store alone during a quiet time

4- Go to a larger store with a friend during a quiet time

3- Go to a small, local store during a busy time

2- Go to a small, local store alone during a quiet time

1- Go to a small, local store with a friend during a quiet time

Figure 7.2 Exposure hierarchy to tackle avoidance.

Facing your fears in this way can temporarily increase your anxiety. We recommend you can use the relaxation exercises described earlier to help you manage any anxious feelings you have about meeting these challenges.

Behavioral Activation

Increasing your activity levels can help to improve low mood. To maintain a sense of well-being, it is important to achieve a balance between pleasurable activities and ones that provide a sense of accomplishment. Often when we feel low, we fall into a pattern of doing less and less. Or we focus on work and chores without allowing ourselves any enjoyable experiences. Unfortunately, this can end up in a downward spiral because we experience fewer pleasurable activities and socialize less, which means that our mood drops even further. We may also become self-critical because it feels like we are not doing or achieving much, which can further affect our mood. One way to tackle this is to keep a diary of your daily activities and, starting from where you are now, gradually introducing more activities. For example, you could add a short walk into your day. You can also make sure there is a good balance of pleasurable and achievement activities. There are apps that can help you to track your activities and rate your mood, and these have been found beneficial in improving low mood.[5] It is important to remember that some days you may not feel like doing these healthy behaviors, and that is okay. Most people report that they do feel better afterward, even if it was hard for them to get started.

The Use of Humor

Stressed Spelled Backwards Is Desserts

While that may seem silly and too simplistic, it may not be such a bad idea to figure out how to turn your stress into positive change through a shift of perspective. Humor is a great way to diffuse tension, and laughter has been shown to have positive effects on overall physical health, psychological well-being, and quality of life.[6] Laughter also reduces stress and muscle tension. Making a commitment to bring it into your life is a good first step.

> Mary notes that even during the most challenging times, through the tears and worry, her family has always found ways to make each other laugh, often at the sheer absurdity of the situations they have found themselves in.

Begin by searching for a few silly items such as pictures, a funny mug, comic strips, or photos of memories that bring you joy or make you giggle. Hang them around your home and/or office. Seek out people who are funny and share your sense of humor, lighten the mood, or make you laugh, and learn a few new jokes that you can try out on others and learn to laugh at yourself. Find a comedian that you can follow and seek out sitcoms or comedies to watch. Smile more and know that at first these changes may seem strange, but with practice they can begin to feel natural.

Give Your Brain a Spa Day

Everyone loves to treat themselves to a spa day, but did you ever consider treating your brain to one? To do so, try combining outdoor (if weather permits) movement with soothing music and then end with a meditation. The activation of the feel-good neurochemicals, the increased blood flow to your brain, and the Vitamin D can make a real difference in how you feel. You can start with just 10 minutes and build up the time slowly if you are able. Try to schedule this each week or, better yet, each day.

When to Seek Further Support

If your symptoms persist or worsen or if attempts to cope lead to unhealthy or unhelpful outcomes, or if you are suffering from red flag symptoms (see below), it is wise to consider getting professional support; we discuss this in more detail in Chapter 10.

Mental Health: Red Flag Symptoms

- Insomnia or hypersomnia (sleeping too much)
- Change in appetite; unexpected weight loss or weight gain
- Suicidal thoughts, self-harm, or risk-taking behaviors
- Angry outbursts or increased irritability
- Alcohol or drug misuse
- Withdrawal from family and friends
- Difficulty focusing or concentrating
- Loss of interest in your favorite activities
- Difficulty controlling or dwelling on repeated thoughts (ruminating)
- Continuing to repeat the same patterns and expecting to achieve new results; feeling "stuck"

8

Maintaining Important Relationships

The people we choose to spend our time with are extremely important to our overall well-being. Healthy social relationships are one of the most important protective factors for our mental health,[1] and they even increase our lifespan.[2] Since social connections are so important to our overall health and well-being, we have dedicated this chapter to exploring how our congenital heart condition (CHC) may impact those connections, for better or worse. We will also discuss ways we can evaluate our relationships and work to sustain, improve, and expand upon them. By gaining an increased awareness and sense of empowerment, it is our hope that you may enjoy having healthy, reciprocal, supportive relationships throughout your lifetime.

Relationship with Yourself

Your relationship with yourself sets the tone for every other relationship that you have.
—Robert Holden[3]

The most important relationship we have is not with our partners, children, friends, or parents, but with *ourselves*. The way we feel about and treat ourselves needs to be considered before we can begin to assess our social interactions and relationships with others. For some people, making this shift in awareness is crucial to understand how your social support system (or lack thereof) may be affecting your mental health, quality of life, and potentially your physical health.

So what exactly does it mean to have a relationship with yourself? It means becoming aware of how you feel about yourself. What are your internal beliefs about who you are as an individual? What is your evaluation of your place in this world? The answers to these questions are connected to your self-esteem.

Self-esteem is the degree to which we accept and value ourselves, thus achieving a basic feeling of self-worth. To have low self-esteem means that you have a negative image of yourself which is global, persistent, and enduring.[4] Negative life experiences, particularly early in life, may lead to the development of an overall negative belief reflecting our sense of worth. Some of the unique health-related challenges faced by those of us with a CHC can negatively impact our self-esteem, leaving us feeling fundamentally "different" from our heart-healthy peers.[5] Being left out or disempowered as a result of our condition may result in feelings of shame, leading to low self-esteem. Low self-esteem can lead to self-criticism and self-defeating behaviors and increase vulnerability to low mood and anxiety. It can also negatively impact relationships. We can work to change this by increasing our awareness and proactively challenging any negative beliefs we hold about ourselves, self-criticism, and self-defeating behaviors while developing a more self-compassionate stance.

Another aspect which influences the relationship we have with ourselves is our self-confidence. Self-confidence is the feeling you have in your ability to accomplish certain tasks or goals. The two are closely related; however, it is possible to have low self-esteem but strong self-confidence. An example of this is someone who knows that she performs well, gets accolades for her ability, but underneath does not like herself, focuses on the negative, and does not feel she deserves the positive attention.

Signs of Low Self-Esteem

- Magnifying negative attributes
- Difficulty saying no and setting appropriate boundaries
- Difficulty expressing your needs
- Putting other people's needs before your own
- Carrying feelings of shame and not feeling worthy
- Negative self-talk, putting yourself down (self-criticism)
- Staying in an unhealthy relationship

- Engaging in self-destructive behaviors
- Filling yourself with status, power, or money

Signs of Low Self-Confidence

- Critical of your abilities
- No confidence or trust in your abilities
- No trust in your judgment
- Magnifying negative attributes
- Negative self-talk
- Unwilling to take on challenges
- Not living up to your potential
- Expect very little out of life

How you feel about yourself is the foundation for all of your other relationships. Self-esteem and self-confidence can affect your thoughts, and this has a domino effect, leading to your emotions, behavior, and ultimately your relationships, as depicted in Figure 8.1.

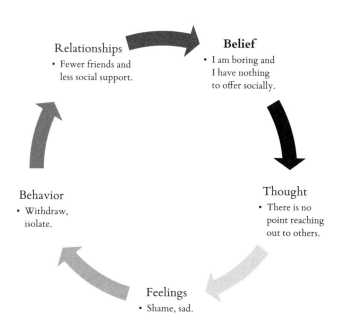

Figure 8.1 Social anxiety vicious cycle.

If this sounds familiar to you, we recommend that you work on both your self-esteem and self-confidence, which in turn will improve your chances of fostering healthy relationships. In addition to the strategies here, you can draw from the techniques covered in Chapter 7 to establish and challenge any negative core beliefs, unhelpful rules for living, self-defeating behaviors, and self-critical thoughts.

Tips for Increasing Your Self-Esteem and Self-Confidence

- Cut out negative self-talk and challenge negative thinking (see Chapter 7).
- Talk to yourself as you would a loved one.
- Realize mistakes happen; don't be so hard on yourself.
- Identify your positive attributes.
- Learn to accept compliments, and acknowledge your successes.
- Treat yourself well.
- Challenge yourself by learning a new skill or trying something different.
- When necessary, begin to set limits with others.
- Cut out or set firm boundaries in toxic relationships.
- Stop comparing yourself to others.
- Stop looking for validation from others.
- Learn to say no.

Replacing Self-Criticism with Self-Compassion

There are many different reasons why we are self-critical. We may have internalized the "voice" of critical parents, bullies, abusers, peers, mentors, and/or social expectations leading to low self-esteem. There are all kinds of reasons why we struggle to be more self-compassionate, including fear of failure and rejection, high standards, low self-worth, and even habit. If you are struggling with self-criticism, you can overcome it and gradually replace it with self-compassion.[6]

Our emotions are controlled and regulated by three systems: the threat, drive, and soothing systems. The *threat system* works to keep us safe by triggering the body's alarm system when we are at risk (as discussed in Chapter 3). As social animals, being excluded from our social group (e.g., by risk of reputation, perceived flaws in our appearance, or feeling different) can trigger this system, leading to feelings of panic, anger, and shame which can lead to self criticism. The second system, our *drive system*, spurs us on to achieve our goals and get things done, providing direction, motivation, and feelings of reward. Finally, our *soothing system* has a calming influence and is linked to feelings of safety and contentment and feeling connected to others. This system is developed in our early years through a healthy attachment to our main caregivers.

As discussed in Chapter 3, if we experience a lot of early adversity, we can develop an overactive *threat system*, whereas interruptions to a secure early attachment can result in an underactive *soothing system*. Some people deal with this by over-relying on their *drive system* to feel good because otherwise the threat system takes over, leading to persistent anxiety or anger. They may find it difficult to activate their soothing system to find peace, calm, and connection (see Figure 8.2).[7]

> *Most survivors, including those who are functioning well—even brilliantly—in some aspects of their lives, face another, even greater challenge: reconfiguring a brain-mind system that was constructed to cope with the worst. Just as we need to revisit traumatic memories in order to integrate them, we need to revisit the parts of ourselves that developed the defensive habits that helped us to survive.*
> —*Bessel van der Kolk,* The Body Keeps the Score[8]

Developing Self-Compassion

The good news is that as adults we can work on nurturing our soothing system through self-compassion and kindness. When you are feeling distress, try the following:

- *Awareness.* Pay attention to the fact that you are experiencing some sort of "suffering" (e.g., emotional pain, mental pain, physical pain).
- *Normalizing.* Recognize that experiencing pain is universal, and it is not your fault or failing, you are not to blame for your pain, and you are not alone in your pain.

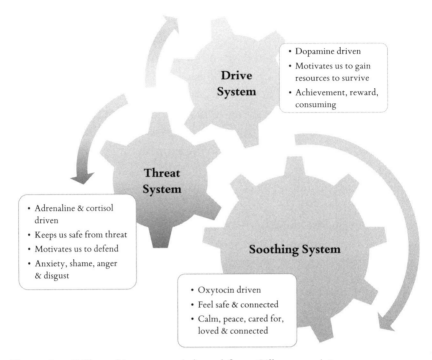

Figure 8.2 Self-soothing system (adapted from Gilbert 2009).[9]

- *Kindness.* Meeting this pain with feelings of kindness, care, warmth, and concern toward yourself.
- *Alleviation.* Focusing your energy on how to alleviate the pain. This may comprise comfort and caring actions, providing a helpful perspective, or finding the strength and courage to take other necessary actions to address the problem being faced.

Challenging Self-Criticism

The opposite of self-compassion is self-criticism, when our threat system is activated. We can also work to minimize this. Some simple but effective steps include the following:

- Start to notice when you are being hard on yourself.
- Instead of just going with what's being said as fact, recognize and label it as an "internal bully." Don't get into an argument with it; try and mindfully observe it and move your attention elsewhere.

- Draw on the techniques in Chapters 5–7 to turn the *threat system* off (such as deep breathing, grounding, and counting to 10).
- Draw on an alternative "self-compassionate voice." If this is a struggle, think about what you would say to a friend, child, or loved one in a similar situation.
- Practice this new way of thinking and this, too, will eventually become a healthy habit.

Self-Compassionate Letter Writing

Writing a compassionate letter to yourself has been found to increase happiness, feelings of self-compassion, and reduce symptoms of depression.[10] If you want to try this out, follow these steps:

- Choose a time when you are unlikely to be disturbed and have peace and calm.
- Identify something that makes you feel ashamed, insecure, or unhappy about yourself. Acknowledge how it makes you feel as honestly as you can.
- Write a letter to yourself expressing compassion, understanding, and acceptance for this part of yourself. It might help to bring to mind someone who loves and accepts you unconditionally, or what you might say to someone else you love unconditionally such as a child.
- In a compassionate way consider the wider context such as your upbringing, challenges you have faced, and other contributing factors.
- Draw from your wisdom to give yourself understanding and advice on how to cope, focusing on constructive changes you can make to manage this perceived flaw. Avoid judging yourself.
- You may want to keep the letter to read the next time you become overwhelmed with self-criticism.

Self-care, self-love, and self-acceptance have helped me deal with my congenital heart disease. I go for monthly massages and take adequate "me" time. I accept my limitations but continue to challenge myself.

—*Lee, 64 years old, United States*

Meditation has also been found to help with increased self-compassion by helping individuals manage stress, anxiety, and chronic pain.[11] Meditation is flexible. There is no time requirement, and it does not require any special equipment. All that is required is an open mind and a quiet space.

One specific meditation that can help increase self-compassion is the *Loving Kindness Meditation*. This meditation can be traced to early Buddhism, and it can be practiced for increased compassion toward self, toward another individual, and/or the greater community, in general. It is a meditation which can invoke feelings of compassion, self-love, kindness, empathy, and warmth. It is one way you can work toward making peace with your body and heart. There are many different versions of this meditation, so if the script that follows doesn't suit you, you may create your own version.

Loving Kindness Meditation

- Create a quiet, private space for yourself. Adjust the temperature and lighting and cut out any possible distractions. Get comfortable and take some deep, controlled breaths, as described in Chapter 5.
- For the initial session, set a timer for 2 minutes (or the amount of time that feels right for you). This will help you to remain focused on your breathing and your intention of increased self-love and compassion. You can, of course, increase the time and build upon it if you decide to practice this each day.
- Imagine someone in your life (past or present) who was kind to you and cared for you unconditionally in a healthy, positive way. This could be a family member, friend, kind empathetic stranger, or beloved pet. Try to visualize that person or pet; breathe in that love and those feelings of empathy, kindness, and acceptance. If you have difficulty identifying someone, then imagine how you would like to be treated, or how you would offer love and kindness to someone in need and turn that feeling onto yourself.
- Repeat the following statements with the intention of increasing those positive, loving feelings within yourself and toward yourself. Continue to breathe deeply and smoothly as you continue to visualize yourself wrapped in the warmth of love and acceptance.

May I be safe and protected
May I experience peace and calm
May I be content and happy
May I be filled with strength and well-being

This might feel strange to you at first, but as you continue this practice it will begin to feel more comfortable and even comforting. If you find it difficult to meditate on your own, there are a number of recordings which offer guided meditations, either online or by downloading a meditation app on your computer or mobile phone.

Change won't happen overnight, but gradually you can turn down the volume on self-criticism while turning up the volume on self-compassion. Once you begin to feel better about yourself, it will be easier to evaluate the other relationships in your life and reach out to increase your social circle, if necessary. Finding and making new friendships happens throughout our life; it is never too late to create new, supportive relationships.

Developing Independence

Understandably, growing up with a serious medical condition can lead to increased dependency on parents and medical care providers, and this can potentially undermine the development of autonomy. Parental overprotection is an understandable and recognized issue for members of this population, adding an additional barrier to achieving independence. Sensitively working toward independence, as possible, will empower you to take charge of your life.

Taking charge of your life will mean different things for different individuals depending on your symptoms, life circumstances, relationships, employment status, and finances. A big piece of moving forward is in your support system and the people in your life. Are you able to handle your healthcare decisions on your own, or do you rely on others to manage your care? Do you have reciprocal and satisfying relationships with family members and friends? Do you have interests or hobbies of your own? Do you have income of your own? There are no right or wrong answers to these questions; this is just an opportunity to reflect and think about whether you are fulfilling your own (realistic) goals.

Relationship with Your Parents or Caregivers

As a parent, I knew I couldn't take away the painful life my baby would endure, but I knew that I had to be with her in hospital to make sure she was as comfortable as she could be and didn't have to wait until a busy nurse had time to sort her pillows or to get her a drink and to stop someone taking her away for yet more painful X-rays when we knew they had already been done. It wasn't just small things; mistakes can and do happen on a very busy short-staffed ward and by being there I could ensure everything was easier for her. I felt like a tiger watching over my cub. In adulthood, her husband has taken on sharing this role when she is in hospital and our family works as a team.

—Elizabeth, parent of an adult with CHC, 72 years old, United Kingdom

Our parents or guardians are our first caregivers and role models. These relationships are the foundation for our emotional development and our future relationships. The hope is that these relationships are positive, loving, and caring. Many individuals with CHC talk about the close bond that occurs as a result of their need to rely on caregivers for physical care and emotional support. As children, we have a basic need to be loved and protected unconditionally, never more so than when we are unwell.[12] Hopefully this is the case for you, and your relationships with your primary caregivers are positive; however, this is not always the case. Sometimes our relationships with our parents are strained due to a number of reasons, including but not limited to mental illness, substance abuse, family distress, or financial stressors.

Developing autonomy and independence is normal and healthy as we become adolescents and young adults. It is normal at this age to want to explore educational and vocational interests and find interests, friends, and loved ones outside of our family circle. Occasionally, that process can be complicated by our CHC or possibly by parental overprotection. A link has been found between posttraumatic stress disorder (PTSD) in parents of children with a CHC and an overprotective parenting style.[13] This connection is understandable, given that our parents are often firsthand witnesses to much of the medical trauma we endure. It makes sense that they want to do whatever is in their power to help us avoid further trauma and protect us at all costs. As a result, they may inadvertently overcompensate in caring for us by "wrapping us up in cotton wool" and micromanaging our lives, limiting our independence by not allowing us to attend events with peers, being overly involved in our lives, and communicating overt acts of sympathy and possibly pity. They may also have lowered expectations of our abilities and not encourage us to challenge ourselves socially, educationally, or otherwise. While understandable, this can contribute to lowered self-confidence, and it passively encourages us to allow our CHC to become the center of who we are as a person, which may lead to a lack of opportunities for education, employment, and social relationships.

*Terri is a 38-year-old woman who has a complex CHC. She had quite a few hospi-
talizations through college and her mid-20s and, as a result, has always lived with her
mother despite dreaming of moving to a place of her own. She was never encouraged to
get a job (even though she has been relatively stable health-wise) and, as a result, does
not have confidence to put herself out there. Her mother still insists on coming into her
cardiology appointments, despite her gentle protest. She would like to be more in control
of her life but is afraid to speak up and unsure of how to take action. She feels helpless
until she asks her team to refer her to a therapist. She works with her therapist on gradually building her confidence and over time gets a part-time job where she makes some
new friends, and eventually she moves into an apartment with one of them. She feels
able to be more assertive with her mother, who recognizes her newfound confidence and
feels more relaxed about letting go.*

If this scenario sounds familiar to you, please know that it is never too
late to make positive changes in your life. Generally a gradual, stepped approach toward increased independence is the best way to proceed. To begin,
a loving but firm talk with your parent/s may be effective at gaining their
support toward this endeavor. Your cardiology care team should be able
to help you to establish realistic expectations in terms of any physical restrictions you may have in relation to activities of daily living and employment. It is through these conversations that you can get a sense of realistic
expectations for your abilities and make a plan to move forward in your
life. Sometimes it may be necessary to employ the help of another family
member, or even a family therapist, to help guide you both through this
process.

Luckily, getting an education today is more accessible with remote classes
and online degree programs. If it is employment you are looking for, sometimes a volunteer position or a part-time job can be a good first step. If you
are unable to work because of your CHC, you might qualify for disability
benefits which may include transportation services, affordable housing, and
home health care. Change is scary, and even positive change can be hard at
first. What matters is that you take and maintain control of your life, so that
you can strive to thrive, to reach your full potential.

Loss of Parent or Caregiver

*At my age I still really miss having my parents around for support. My siblings and
spouse care but don't really get it, and I don't want to burden my child. It's become*

a lonely and scary time of life for me. When you have a CHC, you feel like a scared
little kid at times no matter how old you are.

—Sandra, 59 years old, Canada

Losing a parent or primary caregiver can be very difficult, even when the
relationship is a conflicted one. For those individuals who had a primary
caregiver supporting them through their CHC journey, this loss may be
felt tenfold because they may no longer have that person who understands
and has borne witness to their struggles and journey related to their CHC.
These individuals may have spent a lifetime accompanying you to doctor's
appointments, sitting by your side in the hospital, and being a sounding
board when you needed emotional support. Some individuals have shared
that they always assumed, "I would go (die) first," so when their primary
caregiver (parent, spouse, sibling, grandparent, etc.) dies, or ages, or becomes
ill themselves, it presents them with deep sadness and grief but also with a
secondary loss. They now must learn how to grieve the loss of their loved
one, while also learning to cope with their CHC without that individual's
support and guidance, which can be scary and disorienting.

If this is the case for you, we recommend that you give yourself the time
and the space to process the loss. Through this process it will be necessary
to figure out a "new normal" in relation to your CHC support. Perhaps you
lived (or live with) with this individual, in which case there may be financial
changes that will occur, or depending on your symptoms you may have relied on them to assist you with your activities of daily living. For some it is
the emotional support that is missing in their absence. It will be important
to try to surround yourself with others who can support you in your grief
(see Chapter 4).

Often there is a succession plan in place, and in the best-case scenarios
it has been discussed prior to their death or disability. If that is not the case,
together with other family members or trusted friends, a new plan can be
made to ensure you receive the care that you need. Your adult congenital
heart disease (ACHD) center may be able to get involved, if needed, and
they may be able to recommend home healthcare and/or transportation
services, if needed, or a therapist to help you to figure out how to increase
your emotional support in their absence.

Dating

Telling people about my heart history usually starts with telling them why I have a scar running down my chest. It became more difficult for me in my early 20s, as I started to meet more new people and to date. I have a standard spiel, but I never know how someone will react—scared, loving, indifferent?

—Merideth, 37 years old, United States

Putting yourself out there to meet a romantic companion can be intimidating, even for our heart-healthy peers. It involves being vulnerable and facing the risk of getting hurt. For some individuals with a CHC, they cite additional concerns such as low confidence with regard to their body image, scarring, cyanosis, and physical symptoms or limitations. It is true that there is a real risk of rejection when we begin dating. This is the case for everyone, but for someone with a CHC they wonder if they will ever be able to find someone who will be comfortable getting close to an individual with a serious, chronic illness. While it may be true that not everyone will be able to handle it, there are many others who will see beyond your condition and appreciate you. Some individuals have reported that they believe their partner's scars were beautiful and showed their strength and courage. Others have reported that their spouse felt their CHC made them more special and a better, more rounded person for their experiences. Other partners had expressed a sense of relief that they now could disclose a health-related challenge of their own.

We want you to know that you deserve to find love and happiness and to be treated with respect as much as anyone. While finding the right person may come with additional challenges for those of us with a CHC, it also enables us to filter those who are authentic and decent.

One of the biggest questions we get is how and when to tell a new romantic interest about their CHC. For some, they prefer to be upfront very early on so that they don't get too attached, and others like to take their time and develop a friendship before disclosing their medical situation. There really is no wrong or right answer to this question. You are in control of the information and the pace at which you share it.

Intimate Relationships

When I was an adolescent, I was certain that no one would marry me because of all my scars and physical symptoms. Somehow I was able to put that fear out of my mind as I got older and have now been happily married for over 20 years.

—Alex, 54 years old, United States

Once you find that special someone, communication will be very important. One thing that some individuals have shared is that they feel like they are a burden to their partner because of their CHC. It's important that you talk to your partner about your concerns. A lack of communication can decrease intimacy and create distance in a relationship. Be sure to ask for what you need in the relationship and be prepared to give and take. Finding the right balance is important as you don't want your CHC to become all-consuming.

If your physical symptoms require a lot of assistance from your partner, perhaps they need to schedule time for self-care. If this is the case, the two of you can make a plan for getting another family member or friend to help out when they cannot be there. Everyone takes risks when entering a committed relationship; there are no guarantees that there will not be hardships. Health issues can come up for either of you, at any time, even if your partner was healthy when entering the relationship.

It is important to remember what brought you together in the first place and continue to schedule plans that you both enjoy, as your CHC will allow. Finding other couples to socialize with can also help so that you do not become isolated. It is important that you find ways to have fun together, focusing not on what you *cannot* do, but on what you *can* do. If you run into problems, many find that couples' therapy can be helpful.

The word trigger *may be a bit overused these days but for someone with a CHC, there are real triggers around fear of dying, pain, feeling inadequate, and I try to keep that in mind when my partner is feeling anxious over something that seems insignificant to me.*

—Xavier, spouse, 52 years old, United States

Good communication is essential in maintaining that close relationship, as is physical closeness. Some people with a CHC worry about sexual intimacy, especially following a period of ill health. For most people with a CHC there is no reason why you cannot enjoy an active sex life. Sex is a form of exercise, so this is something we recommend you discuss with your health-care team, particularly following surgery. Make sure to also equip yourself with birth control and sexually transmitted disease (STD) protection infor-mation. Loss of sex drive can be a symptom of anxiety or depression while certain medications can contribute to loss of libido, impotence, and vaginal dryness. If these are concerns for you, we recommend you speak with your nurse, physician, or possible relationship therapist. Try not to be embar-rassed; healthcare professionals are used to answering this kind of question, and you certainly won't be the first (or last) to ask.[14]

Parenting

Growing up with a mom who has CHC has made me never take good health for granted. I know that her health struggles have helped make her the strong mother that she has always been for me and my sister.

—Sedona, 22 years old, United States

Parenting is not only one of the most rewarding jobs; it is also one of the most difficult ones. Having a child is an extraordinary experience, an ex-perience that will change your life forever. It is impossible to know what it will be like until your little one arrives. With the special cuddles and kisses also come late-night feedings, tantrums, and worry. Parenting can be exhausting for even our heart-healthy peers.

For many of us with a CHC, there is an added layer of worry about having the stamina to care for our children not only physically but also emotionally. Some parents express feelings of guilt about not being able to keep up physically with their children, feel sad that they are often fatigued, or wonder if they are a burden because of frequent hospitalizations. It is important to remember that children are extremely resilient, and they will love you no matter what. Parenting with a CHC can be hard, but you can use a lot of what you learned from your illness to be a great parent. Your resilience and wisdom about what is important in life are qualities you can use when dealing with your children. The best gift you can give your chil-dren isn't playing ball with them; it is giving them your unconditional love and acceptance. It takes a village to raise a child, and reaching out to your wider social network for support to ensure all of their needs are met is key to good parenting. One of the most important things is that you surround yourself with a lot of support. If you insist on pushing yourself too hard, you will risk burnout and everyone will suffer. By looking after yourself, being realistic, recognizing your own limits, and asking for help, you will ensure your child enjoys a happy, healthy, full childhood experience.

Talking to Your Child about Your Congenital Heart Condition

Many parents wonder how to talk to their children about their CHC. Understandably they don't want to upset them or needlessly worry them. In reality, for many individuals, their CHC will most likely be a part of our children's lives, whether you talk about it or not. Children can sense when their parents are upset or stressed, even if nothing is said. Your children will likely notice if you are feeling fatigued and unwell, and they will know if you need to be hospitalized. As difficult as it might be for you, being open and gently honest with them is what we recommend. Children are more likely to feel anxious and imagine the worst if they think secrets are being kept from them. They are more likely to experience trauma if they have not been prepared (e.g., if you suddenly need to be hospitalized). These conversations are not easy. There are ways you can be gentle and give information in a contained and age-appropriate manner. What you would say to a 5-year-old will differ from what you tell your 15-year-old.

Modeling gentle honesty, even during painful times, teaches a child about the importance of healthy, loving relationships that they can depend upon. It also communicates that they are an important part of the family.

For most of us, our diagnosis was given the day we were born, or years before our children were born. There is a good possibility that at a very young age, your CHC was an aspect of your family life that was casually talked about as symptoms or hospitalizations came up. If this was the case, your children most likely are aware that you have something wrong with your heart and it may have been talked about over the years. If it hasn't been discussed, we urge you to remember that it is never too late to make a change in the way you handle this with your children. We suggest that you gauge the information you give them depending on the severity of your CHC and on their age. Try to be calm, clear, and loving when you speak to them. Always gauge how they are feeling and what they want to know. While it is important that you keep the door open for their ongoing questions, you don't want to overburden them with too much information. Always encourage them to talk about their feelings to either you or another supportive family member.

Addressing Common Issues That May Arise

The three questions most children will have on their minds are the following[15]:

- *Did I cause this?* Children will think that somehow, something they did may have caused us to have these symptoms/illness or that a change in their behavior might make things okay. They may feel guilty as a result.
- *Can I catch this?* Children may worry that by being with us they can catch a CHC, or that it will be genetically passed on to them.
- *Who will care for me if you die?* Children will want to know who will be there for them if we were to die.

These questions may come up, and if they do not, we still recommend that you address each one. Some of the correct messages to clearly give your children may be as follows:

- *We don't know what caused my CHC, but we know for sure that nothing you did caused this and nothing you may do will ever cause any of my symptoms.*
- *You cannot catch this. A CHC is not contagious; it is not like a cold.* In terms of genetics, most children will have had a fetal echocardiogram done, which can rule out any CHC (if you are connected genetically). If your child is not connected to you genetically and they are concerned, we suggest you speak with their pediatrician to ease their worry.
- For the third question, if this comes up, you will need to give it some thought and make a plan. Do you have a will? Who would be their guardian should something happen to you? Is there another parent involved? They may ask what would happen if both of you died. You may want to go into some detail as appropriate, depending on the age of your children. The key message is that while this is very unlikely to happen, you will make sure that there will always be someone to take care of them.

Finding a trusted confidant to talk to about your challenges is essential. However, that person should never be your child, no matter what their age. Using your child as your emotional support will only burden them with worry. One of our main roles as parents is to "emotionally contain" our child's distress.[16] This means providing them with a safe space to express their feelings by staying calm and collected. By "holding" their difficult emotions and effectively modeling self-soothing and coping, children learn how to regulate their emotions.[17] It is our job to show them that together we can cope with whatever life throws at us.

Your child may also benefit from their own confidant. They may want to talk to other trusted adults about how they are feeling, and that's okay. Perhaps it is their other parent, an aunt, special teacher, or counselor; what's important is that you both have people who will be there for you. This is especially important if you are facing hospitalization, surgery, or a more acute period of illness.

Friends and Relatives

My sister was often in the children's hospital which was always a worrying time for the family. Later in life it has been even more worrying as adult care does seem less consistent. As a sibling of such a special person, it does inspire resilience within oneself which is useful through all of life's challenges.

—Brother, 47 years old, United Kingdom

Friends and relatives can be a great source of security, love, and fun. We look to our family and friends for comfort and support when we are not feeling well or during a medical crisis. Yet dealing with ongoing health issues can alter some of these relationships. Perhaps your family isn't as sensitive to your health-related experiences as you would have hoped. Or maybe your good friend is upset because you have had to cancel the last few plans you had with her due to your fatigue or you feel let down because she didn't visit or offer support during a period of hospitalization. It may be that you sense a sibling feels resentful of the attention your condition gets without grasping your suffering. If you are finding that an important relationship is strained or if you are not feeling supported by those around you, rather than pushing them away or bottling everything up, try to speak with them about your feelings and ask for what you need while being open to their needs, too. Your connections with loved ones are important. Having healthy relationships requires both individuals to devote equal time and attention to each other.

When we became friends, it quickly became clear how much she has to juggle and bal-ance on a daily basis due to her CHC. I realized that activities that I take for granted are not always as straightforward for her.

—Friend, 45 years old, United Kingdom

Some individuals hold back in sharing their struggles for fear of creating worry in their loved ones, or they are afraid that they may become a burden. It is important to remember that our good friends and close family want to be there for us. Close relationships are built on sharing, intimacy, and trust. By showing your vulnerability during hard times, your family or friends will be more likely to open up to you when they are struggling. Expecting our loved ones to "mind-read" what is going on for us can lead to frustra-tion, misunderstanding, and seldom leads to us getting our needs met.

It is important to know that friendships change throughout our lives. This is also true for our heart-healthy peers. It can be difficult to watch as a friendship fizzles out. This can sometimes occur when the two of you don't have as much in common anymore. This can also occur if either of you is not getting your needs met and, after talking about it, the dynamic still doesn't change. Some other common concerns individuals with CHCs cite and some possible solutions are depicted in Table 8.1.

One very important element in feeling better physically is keeping strong, healthy relationships to those close to you. It is important to re-member that your CHC may affect each member of your family and that keeping those relationships close requires both individuals to make ongoing efforts. Always remember to let those important to you know how you feel about them. Let them know how important they are to you, how proud of them you are, or how much you appreciate all they are to you, if that is in fact how you feel.

In reality, relationships can also be hard work. There are occasional argu-ments and times that we may need to compromise. Some situations even call for taking a break from each other, only to come back together again once we've had some space and gained some perspective. It is important to recognize when the relationship stress is no longer normal, or when the relationship is becoming toxic, or even abusive. If the relationship is abu-sive in any way, emotionally, sexually, or physically, then the relationship

Table 8.1 Dealing with Friendship Challenges

Friendship Challenge	Possible Solution or Alternative View
"I am afraid to let my friends know about my CHC for fear of being treated differently."	You are in charge of when and who to tell about your CHC. Once trust is established, it is easier to let them know about your CHC and about this fear of being treated too delicately.
"People don't believe me when I am feeling unwell, and they express doubt when I need to set a limit."	Share your feelings with them and educate them about your CHC and the reasons for your symptoms. If they continue to question you, consider whether this friendship is a healthy support or if it is becoming too stressful.
"Maybe I am being overly sensitive to my friends' comments and behavior."	Ask yourself: Are you often defensive? Do you take things too personally? Could you be misinterpreting your friends' lack of availability as being aloof to the friendship when actually they are dealing with troubles of their own? If the answer to all is no, then have a talk with them about how their comments and behavior make you feel. If there isn't a change, then the relationship may need to be re-evaluated.
"My friend treats me with kid gloves."	Ask yourself: Is this their personality? Do they treat everyone this way? Am I giving off vibes that I am helpless? If the answer to both questions is no, speak with them. Let them know you value that friendship and promise to let them know when and if you need help.
"I am being left out."	If you feel like you are being left out, then have a talk with them about why this is happening and how you feel. If this continues, it may be time to re-evaluate the friendship.
"My friend makes 'jokes' about my condition that are actually hurtful, but I just laugh along."	It is important to tell friends when they have crossed a line. It is only funny if you are both amused.

needs to be ended for your own safety and well-being. Some relationship dynamics are not as clear cut, as in the case of those that may be deemed toxic. A toxic relationship is one that is not supportive and caring; it is not built on trust and kindness. It is a relationship that may be stressful and full of conflict. These relationships can be emotionally harmful. Some examples include the following:

• Being taken advantage of repeatedly
• Always giving and not getting anything in return

- Dishonesty and jealousy
- Frequent arguing
- Being criticized, put down, and told you're "oversensitive" if you challenge them
- Feeling like you are "walking on eggshells" and the relationship is unpredictable

This may also be a reason to end the relationship. You deserve to have relationships that are healthy, caring, and supportive. Relationships should be an equal give and take, and you should be getting back from your friendships/relationships what you give. You should be having more good times than bad times.

> I found someone else at work who has a CHD, and she and I bonded immediately. It was like meeting someone else who speaks my native language after years and years of not knowing anyone else that spoke that language.
>
> —Lenae, 33 years old, United States

Even our closest family and friends may find it difficult to fully understand what we are experiencing. Some individuals with CHCs find that speaking with a peer with similar experiences can be helpful. Finding a peer mentorship program, online support group, or being connected with another CHC patient through your ACHD specialized care center can be extremely helpful in feeling heard and supported.

Developing Healthy Communication and Boundaries

> Our greatest freedom is our freedom to choose our attitude.
>
> —Viktor Frankl[18]

Healthy adult relationships are reciprocal and respectful with appropriate boundaries. The key to getting our needs met and communicating them effectively is to develop a healthy, adult, assertive style and to surround ourselves with others who are also able to communicate in this way, as possible. Poor communication can damage our relationships and prevent us from getting our needs met. This might include blaming, shaming, passive aggression, sarcasm, and game playing. Good communication is a skill we can learn.

Simple Steps to Better Communication

- Try not to be reactive; step away from the conversation if it is getting heated.
- Try not to start a sensitive conversation on an empty stomach, when you are tired, or after one of you has been drinking alcohol.
- Give yourself time and space to consider what you want to communicate and how to say this calmly.
- Listen to what the other person is really saying, too, and try and not make assumptions. Check in with them if you need to clarify: "Are you saying . . .?" or "Do you mean . . . ?"
- Use "I feel" rather than "You are" statements because when we start accusing, the other person immediately goes on the defensive.
- Try not to communicate over social media or text when feeling upset. It is much easier to misunderstand each other when not speaking directly to one another. If you have to keep it to email or text, try to wait 24 hours before responding.

There are four main styles of communication (as depicted in Figure 8.3). Assertive communication skills help to get your perspective across in a clear, honest, and direct way while taking into account the other person's view. This healthy type of communication is based on mutual respect, and it lets people know how you honestly feel, in a productive, calm, and kind

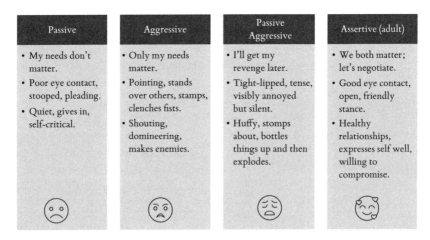

Passive	Aggressive	Passive Aggressive	Assertive (adult)
• My needs don't matter. • Poor eye contact, stooped, pleading. • Quiet, gives in, self-critical.	• Only my needs matter. • Pointing, stands over others, stamps, clenches fists. • Shouting, domineering, makes enemies.	• I'll get my revenge later. • Tight-lipped, tense, visibly annoyed but silent. • Huffy, stomps about, bottles things up and then explodes.	• We both matter; let's negotiate. • Good eye contact, open, friendly stance. • Healthy relationships, expresses self well, willing to compromise.

Figure 8.3 Communication styles.

way. Assertiveness is about recognizing that we each have different wants and needs and working together to negotiate a compromise, rather than demanding that you get your own way or easily subjugating to another. Being assertive isn't always easy, especially if you are used to overly pleasing people, communicating passively, or if you tend to have a temper. However, this style can help you to authentically express a wide range of feelings which can enhance your self-esteem. Of course, none of these styles will guarantee that you will get what you want, but this is a way to openly and maturely express yourself while maintaining healthy relationships and minimizing the chances of hurting others.

What Assertive Communication Might Look Like

- Explaining to others that you may not be able to commit to something because you are unsure how you will feel
- Letting others know that you will need to take rest breaks
- Explaining to others you may not be able to take part in certain events or will only be able to participate for a shorter period of time (e.g., "I will come along for the meal")
- Letting others know your health affects you and asking them for their understanding
- Assertively correcting others if they make wrong assumptions or say things that are unhelpful, negative, or discriminatory
- Asking for a meeting with your manager to discuss how your condition impacts you and negotiating how to make your workload manageable

Dealing with Unhelpful Positivity

Unhelpful or toxic positivity is when someone minimizes or denies your experiences with overly optimistic "feel good" quotes or statements. Often these comments shut down any opportunity to open up about how you are really feeling or discuss the difficulties you face. They can leave you feeling invalidated, silenced, and alone in your experience. This can also build up resentment in relationships with your loved ones or healthcare professionals.

Some common examples include the following:

- You're lucky you can cope so well. I hate hospitals.
- You're so brave; it's nothing to you.
- I guess you must be used to it.
- But you look so well.
- Other patients don't experience that; I am sure it is nothing.
- I've seen a lot worse.
- Everything happens for a reason.
- Look on the bright side.
- Happiness is a choice.
- You should be grateful.
- You're lucky to be alive.
- It can't be that bad; you manage to (work/go out/shop).
- Good job you can cope so well; I couldn't deal with it.
- I get tired, too. Everyone does. You've just gotta keep pushing through it!

   If this is a pattern that you have noticed in some of your relationships, then you can try to kindly but firmly address it by explaining how these comments make you feel and what you need to feel supported. Some people genuinely do not know what to say and struggle with being empathic, so they fall back on trite phrases or quotes without realizing the impact (they may even regret it later). By telling them what you would like from them (a hug, validation, just to listen or sit with you), your relationship will deepen. It is important to not let this kind of response silence you. You deserve to be supported through your experiences, and finding people who are able to tolerate and validate the reality and not just the "brave," "inspirational" stoic you is essential to this.

Build Your Team

Building Your Team Exercise

We all have different needs, including emotional, practical, intellectual, and fun, that can't be met by just one person. As such, it's healthy to have a network of different people[19] with realistic expectations about what each relationship can offer. The aim of this exercise is to explore whether your current network meets all of your needs.

Get a piece of paper and write your name in the middle; then draw lines representing how close you feel to each significant person in your life, adding their name at the end of the line; this may end up looking a bit like a spider (with you as the body). You can then add information beside each name, including how often you are in contact, what kind of support they offer you, and how long you have known them. Consider whether your social needs are currently being met. Is there scope to develop and nourish some relationships? Is it time to add boundaries to others? Are these relationships reciprocal; how do you feel after you have spent time together? What changes would help you meet your needs? (see Figure 8.4).[20]

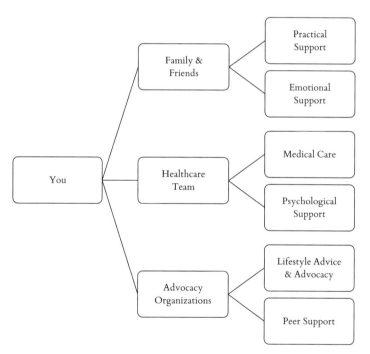

Figure 8.4 Social support network.

9

Coping with Medical Procedures, Events, and Symptoms

Living with a congenital heart condition (CHC) can involve dealing with uniquely challenging medical procedures and events beyond that of our family and friends, yet we are not given a handbook on how to deal with them practically, physically, or emotionally. Often, it is assumed we are "used to" facing these challenges, when in reality it can be more difficult for us because of the reminders of difficult past experiences in the hospital and the challenges we may face in the future. It is unusual to have to face the same potentially traumatizing experiences repeatedly, especially from childhood, with the knowledge you will likely face them again. It is important to remember that as adults we have more control about what is happening to us than we had as children. While there can be difficult experiences we must face, it is important to acknowledge and recognize any normal emotional response to this (just because you have no choice doesn't mean you aren't allowed a reaction). There are many things that can help to psychologically prepare us for these medical challenges. These may include becoming an "expert patient" by understanding our condition and why medical procedures are required, what to expect during them, and the expected recovery time. Further, strategies for managing discomfort, pain, and medical events (e.g., emotional release, relaxation techniques, and distraction); developing a positive outlook (e.g., positive imagery, self-compassion, and thought challenging); managing our emotions (emotional regulation); communicating our needs assertively; and accessing social support are all protective factors, too.[1]

We want you to be fully equipped with all the skills and information you may need to help mitigate the impact of any medical adversities. As such, in this chapter we will consider the medical side of living with a CHC, including the most common cardiac procedures, surgeries, and medical challenges and how to cope with them.

Self-Management: Embrace Being an Expert Patient

In many ways, living with a CHC is a bit like being an Olympic athlete. Every day we push our bodies to the limit, so we need to take lots of care of ourselves to reach our fullest potential. This is why proactively maintaining your general health and well-being as best you can through self-care is essential before, during, and after any medical procedures. Have the confidence to listen to your body, recognize your limits and strengths, and treat yourself with self-compassion and acceptance.

You are an essential partner in your healthcare team, and it is vital that you are taken seriously, listened to, and validated by your healthcare providers. As such, it is important that you have a cardiology team that you trust and feel you can partner with. There is a saying that "informed patients live longer." As an expert patient, it is important to have as good an understanding of your condition as possible or for you to have an advocate that does.

> ER (emergency room) visits always leave me exhausted, both physically and emotionally. It took me a long time to realize that a lot of medical professionals don't know the first thing about ACHD (adult congenital heart disease). I remember once I went to the ER with chest pain and blue fingertips. I had to wait in the ER for 12 hours until they finally saw me. The doctor who saw me acted odd, as though he didn't believe me when I explained my symptoms. He even told me he was going to send me home—without being seen by the ACHD team at the hospital. Fortunately his attending physician came in and told him absolutely not, that I needed to be kept overnight for observation, and then be seen by my ACHD team in the morning.
>
> —Lenae, 33 years old, United States

It can help to have a summary copy of your medical notes and care plan in case you end up in Accident and Emergency (or the emergency room), especially if you are out of the area on vacation or otherwise. It is also useful to have a copy of what a normal electrocardiogram (ECG) is for you. It is wise to plan ahead for emergencies by keeping numbers of key contacts. Sharing all of this essential information with loved ones is important. Depending on your condition and your personal choice, you may want to wear a talisman or MedicAlert necklace or bracelet to indicate your condition and emergency contact numbers to others in the event of an emergency, or you may choose to store this information on an app in your mobile phone. Some people store emergency numbers under "ICE" (in case of emergency) in their phone.

Accessing the Right Care

I have supreme confidence in my cardiologist, and we have frank discussions regarding my CHD. Much of my appointment-related stress throughout the years has involved the cardiac fellows or residents that examine me prior to my cardiologist's appearance. I find myself playing strong defense against their questions and not opening up until the cardiologist is there to guide the conversation and any subsequent need for care.

—Mitch, 59 years old, United States

As previously discussed, many adults throughout the developed world with a CHC are not under the care of a specialist congenital cardiology service for a variety of reasons. For example, in the United States, it was found that only 10% of those CHC patients who could benefit from ACHD care end up receiving it.[1] This is concerning since one study showed that being connected to specialized ACHD care was crucial to reducing the risk of mortality.[2]

In the early days there was no "specialist" care. Often a general cardiologist took a special interest in congenital cases, perhaps because they came across an interesting or needy case and decided to "have a go." The specialist field of congenital cardiology is now established, and there is no longer any need for this to happen. It is recognized internationally that care of people with a CHC should be under the guidance of a specialist trained to provide care to congenital cardiac patients.[3] Internationally, healthcare guidelines recommend meeting with an ACHD-accredited program at least once.[4] Fortunately, there are now also two sets of written guidelines which indicate the level of care patients should receive depending upon their diagnosis and symptoms. They are the American Heart Association/ American College of Cardiology (AHA/ACC) and the European Society of Cardiology Guidelines for Management of Adults with Congenital

Heart Disease.⁵ Not all nonspecialist healthcare providers are aware of these recommendations, and you might meet resistance in trying to gain a referral to specialist care, but it is important to advocate for yourself.

If you live in the United States or other countries with private healthcare systems, having health insurance is very important. In the United States, the Affordable Care Act (2010) made it possible for health insurance to be attainable based on lower-cost policies, with no pre-existing condition exclusions, and extended parental insurance to dependent offspring until age 26. This provided vital options to the young adult CHC community and kept many from being lost to follow-up based on lack of insurance coverage.

> I have learned to take charge of my health and be my own health advocate. In the past, I just blithely accepted any doctor the practice assigned to me. In a few cases I just didn't feel the doctor was right for me. It was a difficult process, but I changed physicians and could not be happier. I am getting the care I need and deserve.
>
> —Lee, 64 years old, United States

You are also entitled to move healthcare providers if you feel that you are not getting the care you need or to ask for a second opinion. Some individuals are hesitant to seek a second opinion for fear of angering or hurting their cardiologist's feelings, yet second opinions are common nowadays and most doctors will understand and appreciate your ability to advocate for yourself. One research study, based in the United States, showed that 21% of patients in the general population who sought a second opinion left with a completely new diagnosis and 66% had their diagnosis better defined or redefined.⁶ CHCs can be complicated and often require advanced training and treatments. It is also important to know that not all hospitals have the same level of skill or have the same technology or surgical equipment.

Knowledge Is Power: Understanding Your Medical Care

> I have found that the best way to advocate for myself has been to equip myself with knowledge. I do this by gathering current information on issues concerning my body, which helps me feel like I've earned a seat at the table when discussing my care with my medical team.
>
> —Lauren, 27 years old, United States

Studies have shown that being psychologically prepared for medical care benefits our physical, psychological, and emotional health.[7] Often when we are staying in the hospital or attending an appointment, we feel disempowered, overwhelmed, and struggle to take things in. We might not feel able to ask even basic questions. Here we have provided a basic summary of what cardiac care can entail. Of course, we are all different, and this very much depends on your condition, but you can use this as a reference to make sense of your own experience. If you think this may be triggering for you, please skip this section.

The Congenital Cardiology Medical Team

When you have a CHC, there will likely be various healthcare professionals involved in your care. It is useful to know what roles they play in helping you manage your condition; they may include those listed in Figure 9.1.

 ACHD Specialist / Congenital Cardiologist: A medical doctor with specialist expertise in congenital cardiac conditions who usually takes charge of your care.

 Anesthesiologist: Doctors with specialist training in anaesthesia, intensive care medicine, and pain management

Cardiac Electrophysiologist: A healthcare professional who is trained in medical physics with expertise in pacemaker and ICD interrogation.

 Cardiac Radiographer: A medical technician who operates equipment to take radiographic images such as X-rays.

 Cardiac Physiotherapist: A person qualified to treat disease or injury by physical methods such as massage, heat treatment, and exercise.

 Cardiothoracic Surgeon: A surgeon who has specialist training and experience in heart and lung surgeries.

Interventional Cardiologist: A cardiologist with additional training in interventional cardiac procedures such as catheterization.

 Psychologist/Counsellor/Clinical Social Worker (US): Someone with professional training and clinical skills to help people learn to cope more effectively with life issues and mental health problems.

 Specialist Congenital Cardiac Nurse: A nurse who specializes in congenital cardiac conditions.

Figure 9.1 Cardiac team.

Cardiac Diagnostic Tests

We have listed the most common types of cardiac procedures used for diagnosis and monitoring in Figure 9.2. Only some of them will apply to you, depending on your condition.

Types of Cardiac Surgery/Procedures

There are various types of surgery or medical procedures that people with a CHC may require, depending on the nature of their condition. Some types of surgery are more invasive than others. You can ask your medical team for more information about any procedures that you require. Some people like more detail than others, and this is completely up to you. Just let your team know how much information is helpful to you.

 Cardiac Catheterization: During this procedure, a thin, flexible tube called a catheter is put into a vein in the groin or neck and threaded through to the heart to provides a 3-D picture. Sedation is used.

 Chest X-Ray: A painless test that takes a photo of the inside of the body.

 Echocardiogram (echo): A painless test that uses sound waves (ultrasound) to create a moving picture of the heart. This allows the medical professional to see the structure of the heart.

 Electrocardiogram (ECG): A painless test that allows the healthcare professional to see the heart's electrical activity.

 Home Monitor: A home monitoring device that "speaks" to the pacemaker or ICD and automatically provides basic information about the cardiac condition and device. It can wirelessly transmit diagnostic information to a service center.

 INR Self-Testing Kit: Allows patients receiving treatment to prevent blood clots to use a self-care app to self-test safely and conveniently their INR levels.

 Pacemaker Interrogation: Painless, non-invasive procedure where a cardiac physician uses a specialist machine to connect, via a magnet and leads, to the pacemaker or ICD. Provides information about how the device is functioning, battery life, and the heart's activity. The settings or parameters of the device can be altered to optimize it.

 24-Heart Monitor: A painless portable monitor which measures heart activity over a specified time so that the healthcare team can look at the recorded information and see how the heart is working.

Figure 9.2 Cardiac procedures.

Social Support

Social support is one of the most protective factors for our mental health and well-being. During medical experiences the soothing presence of a loved one has particular health benefits across the lifespan.[8] Research studies show that soothing touch expresses compassion and provides feelings of safety and comfort,[9] with one study finding that preterm babies gain more weight when they are touched.[10] Human contact is so important that "skin-to-skin" contact or "kangaroo care" has been shown to reduce mortality, illness, infection, length of hospital stay, sleep issues, and pain in preterm babies.[11] Compassion is also expressed through vocalization,[12] such as the soothing voice of a partner, parent, or friend. One recent study found that the mother's voice can decrease pain and increase oxytocin levels in preterm infants during painful procedures.[13] As such, it can really make a significant difference to reach out to loved ones and, for example, ask them to accompany you to hospital appointments or visit you during hospital stays. Bringing a close family member or friend with you to hospital appointments can also help you to remember any new care instructions or recommendations that may be provided them a better understanding of what is going on.

> *Most adults with congenital heart disease (CHD) have become conditioned to living with their CHD alone, simply because that's the only way they know. Quite simply, it does not have to be like this. Facebook alone has opened the world to adults with CHD to connect. Never before have there been opportunities to reach out and connect with other CHD adults than there is today. Social media has changed the landscape. With connection, there is belief. With connection there is understanding. With connection comes support, from the only group of people who truly understand. If this resonates with you, reach out. Connect. You will never regret it. Don't be alone.*
>
> —*Stuart, 55 years old, New Zealand*

Talk It Out

Studies show that if you prepare emotionally for surgery, you will have less pain and recover more quickly.[14] Having a safe space to explore and share your feelings is key to this. This might involve speaking to a close friend, family member, a sympathetic nurse, or if available a counselor or mental health professional. It is okay to cry, have a bit of a rant, and get all of your feelings out. If you don't feel like talking to anyone about how you are feeling, it might help to write it down in a diary or notebook instead. A growing number of CHC centers have a mental health practitioner with whom you can connect, or you may be able to speak to a specialist nurse. Some hospitals provide alternative or holistic services to help you prepare emotionally. If you would like to speak with someone about this and your CHC center does not have these resources, ask your healthcare team if they can recommend a mental health professional in the community.

When Aimee found out that she needed another surgery, she became extremely anxious. She asked her CHC doctor if he could recommend alternative treatments to help prepare her emotionally for surgery. He did not know of any but offered to research. Two days later a clinical social worker called her and offered telephone sessions to help her feel more relaxed before surgery. They scheduled a few remote counseling sessions to practice breathing and visualization exercises, which she used on her way into surgery and really helped.

Preparing for Medical Appointments

Spending time in the hospital for appointments, procedures, or surgery can understandably be a difficult and stressful time. Go easy on yourself and look after yourself as much as possible. Little things can make a big difference. Appreciate that this is a difficult experience and that it is understandable if you get upset at times or feel anxious, angry, or down. This does not mean that you are not coping, just that you are a normal human being who is reacting to exceptionally difficult circumstances with normal emotions.

Assertive communication (Chapter 8) will better enable you to share your feelings (e.g., anxious, scared, or frustrated) and ask your care team for assistance. It may help to organize an extra meeting with the surgeon, doctor, or specialist nurse if you have additional questions about the upcoming procedure or surgery. It is common to revert to the "patient role" during medical consultations. Many people report feeling anxious and disempowered during these encounters and find it difficult to articulate what they want to say. This is even more common if you have had difficult experiences previously with healthcare professionals or traumatic medical experiences. It can help to make a list of your questions beforehand. Take a notepad with you so you can also make a note of their answers. You may also want to take someone with you such as your partner, a family member, or a trusted friend for support and also to act as a backup "memory." It is useful to ask how you can reach your CHC team, if needed, should you have additional questions or concerns after your appointment.

If you have had difficult medical experiences in the past that make your care more challenging or evoke strong distressing feelings, then you can inform your healthcare team about this. You can ask them to write this in your medical notes so that additional care, support, and time are provided for any procedures you find particularly difficult. For example, if you have a needle phobia, you can ask to be referred to a therapist for treatment. Following this you can ask for additional time, support, and, if it helps, to be lying down before blood is taken and additional recovery time afterward. If you generally find coming to the hospital more challenging, you can tell your healthcare team this so they can better understand how you're feeling. If there are particular things that you find helpful, then you can explain this to them and ask for your needs to be taken into consideration. This may include having your partner present during appointments, having a consistent point of contact, seeing the same consultant at appointments, being provided with a care plan in event of emergency, and being copied into any medical letters about you. If you have a complex medical history and have experienced medical trauma, this should be taken into consideration by your healthcare team and dealt with sensitively and compassionately. We have provided guidance for healthcare professionals in Chapter 12, which you may want to share with your team.

Preparing for Time in the Hospital: Assemble Your Team

If you are going to be spending time in the hospital, it can be useful to give a list of your key contacts to a chosen individual and ask them to give updates, if needed. The people on this list may include your loved ones, neighbors, and any physician involved in your CHC care. Communicate with them about what is going on and how they can be helpful.

Many patients have said they have a hard time doing this, as they "don't want to ask for help or be a burden." However, it is likely that your family and friends want to be there for you, and it will make it easier for them if you let them know how to help you best. Asking for help can also create more closeness in a relationship and that "helper" will be more likely to ask you for help in the future, if needed.

Self-Care in the Hospital: Preparing for Surgery or Invasive Medical Procedures

If you have time before being admitted to the hospital, we suggest packing a bag with all of the "physical tools" that can help you get through this difficult experience. Take things that make you feel better, such as photographs of loved ones and happy times, music that you find comforting, comfortable nightwear (PJs that button up are easier to take on and off; after cardiac surgery it can be painful to lift your arms up to put a top over your head), body cream that you like the smell of, a small handheld fan, a pillow and favorite blanket, games to play (electronic or playing cards), a good book, your toiletries/toothbrush, your favorite sweets, and a new "going home" outfit. It is wise to hand over any items of jewelry, your wallet, house and car keys, or other valuable items to a family member or friend to keep safe. Please note that if you are going to be staying in intensive care, you may not be able to take any personal items with you. In this case you may want to give this bag to a loved one to bring to the hospital once you are back on the main ward.

Coping during Surgery and Medical Procedures

Samantha dreaded the day when she needed to have her pacemaker replaced again. She was so surprised when it ended up being much easier than what she had remembered from her last surgery 8 years earlier.

Going for surgery can make you feel lots of mixed emotions. In addition to feeling hopeful, it is normal to feel anxious, frightened, down, angry, and upset. Fear and anxiety are the body's normal response to a threat. Even when you understand that you need surgery to survive, it is difficult to override the body's instinctive response to being hurt. The nature of the doctor/nurse–patient relationship can also lead to you feeling disempowered. However, understanding why you feel like this and learning how to better manage these feelings can make this difficult time a little easier and make you feel more in control of what is happening to you.

We recommend that you draw from the strategies or "emotional tools" described in Chapters 5–7 as often as you need—at home or in the hospital. Distraction, grounding, breathing, and relaxation exercises are useful for dealing with pain, discomfort, and overwhelming feelings of anxiety or distress. Tasks that focus attention without requiring too much thought are good for distracting an agitated mind. Repetitive tasks such as playing simple card games like patience, solitaire, or snap or puzzles such as sudoku or a crossword might help. Other ways to distract yourself include watching a favorite movie, listening to music, knitting, or chatting with loved ones.

Thought challenging (see Chapter 7) may be useful if you find you are catastrophizing or ruminating. You can draw on the techniques for self-compassion (see Chapter 8) if you find yourself becoming self-critical, while assertiveness techniques will help you communicate your needs with healthcare providers and loved ones.

Drawing from emotional regulation techniques (see Chapter 6) to acknowledge your feelings may also help. Let your doctor know if you are struggling with excessive anxiety, insomnia, or depression. If needed, they may be able to refer you to a mental health professional to speak to with the goal of feeling more prepared emotionally.

Sometimes individuals are admitted to the hospital right from their cardiologist's office. Other times they are able to go home and arrive back at the hospital the night before or the morning of the surgery. Once admitted, if there are any questions or concerns, then speak to your ACHD team about them. If they are unavailable, then ask a nurse. If they are unable to answer your concern, request that they contact your doctor. You know your body better than anyone, and your concerns should always be heard. If you do not understand what is happening to you, then ask. If you are not satisfied with the answer, then ask to speak to someone else. Be polite and reasonable but assertive (it is easy to become frustrated and angry, but this won't get you the reaction that you want). You may want to ask a family member to help you advocate for yourself if you are having difficulty getting what you need.

Pre-Surgery/Pre-Procedure

Prior to surgery you will usually be asked to fast (not eat) for 8 hours. You will usually get to meet the surgeon and anesthesiologist beforehand and be asked to sign a consent form. If you have any particular questions, then you have the right to ask these of your medical team. It is your body, and you have the right to know as much as you feel comfortable with. It is a good idea to write your questions down before meeting with them so that you don't forget them. Don't worry about appearing silly; it is okay to ask for things to be explained clearly. Ask them to draw a diagram if that would help you to understand. Some other pre-surgery tips include the following:

- Find out what time your surgery will happen, how long it will take, and the likely recovery time needed so that you can prepare yourself and make plans for recovery.
- Find out what is likely to happen when you come around from the anesthetic. Will you be kept in the recovery room? Will you be going to an intensive care ward or the routine cardiac ward? Will you be attached to a ventilator, drip, or catheter? You can feel disoriented after surgery, and it will help if you can make sense of where you are and what is going on.
- What is likely to be the impact of surgery on your body? For example, do bones need to be broken? How long will it take to heal?
- If you are worried about pain, ask how this will be managed.
- If you want numbing cream prior to getting a cannula or intravenous therapy (IV), ask for it. It isn't always offered to adults, but there is no reason why you can't have it.
- If anesthesia usually makes you nauseous, then you can be given medication before surgery to stop this from happening. Discuss this with the anesthesiologist beforehand.
- If you have concerns about scars, ask about this. It takes time to come to terms with a new scar, but this process is easier if you are prepared and know what to expect.
- If you want to know, then ask about the risks involved. This way you can prepare yourself for any realistic outcome. Often when we don't know the facts, it is easier to imagine the worst.
- Think about whether you would like to make a living will and organize this with a lawyer beforehand. In the United States an advance directive can often be completed during hospital admissions. We recommend you request the forms beforehand so that you have time to think about the different scenarios and decide if you would like to appoint a healthcare proxy, or individual in charge of your healthcare. This document outlines your wishes should anything unexpected happen during the surgery and you become incapacitated.

- If you have a few weeks to prepare before the surgery, try to stay healthy by staying away from anyone who might be ill and have a conversation with your doctor about any restrictions on your physical activity.
- Talk to your doctor about the medications you are taking and if and when to discontinue them. It is important to be completely honest with your doctor so there are no risks of drug interactions.
- Often patients are placed in a shared room. If you prefer a private room, request it before and also during your admission process. Depending on the hospital's census that day, it may or may not be possible.
- The night before surgery you might be offered a sleeping pill and on the day you may or may not be offered premedication, which is usually made up of sedatives to try and help you feel calmer before going to the theater/operating room. It is up to you if you want to take these.
- Plan to have someone stay in the hospital (if allowed) or request a visitor accommodation for the first night in case you need extra assistance.
- Plan your transportation after discharge.
- Put a plan in place for household help and meals. Ask a friend or family member to organize meals for when you get home.

Visualize Your Recovery

Visualization can be a powerful tool for healing. Research has shown that guided imagery not only reduces anxiety in many patients going in for cardiac surgery, but it can also decrease their length of stay in the hospital and decrease pain after surgery.[15] Research at Harvard University has shown that visualization can increase an individual's immunity,[16] which can only help in the healing process.

The imagination is a powerful tool that can help us through difficult times. For instance, if we imagine sad things happening to us, we will begin to feel unhappy. If we think anxious thoughts, we will begin to feel anxious. Therefore, as we are gearing up for our surgery, imagining healing and positive images will help us to feel calmer and more relaxed beforehand. Preparing for surgery emotionally has been shown to decrease our pain and recovery time.[17] *The key is to focus on the positive outcome of your surgery, rather than on the surgery itself.* It takes just as much energy to worry about the worst scenario as it does to picture the best possible outcome. If you are able to practice this twice a day leading up to your surgery, it will most likely be more effective when using it at the hospital.

You may begin to practice this exercise whenever you find out you need to have surgery. It may feel unnatural at first, but as time progresses it will hopefully begin to feel more comfortable, and even soothing. If you don't have a lot of time to prepare before surgery, that is okay; this can still be effective. Some people find this visualization helpful the day of surgery, while waiting in the pre-op room.

Visualization Exercise

- Get comfortable; if possible adjust the temperature in your room or use a blanket if needed. Begin to practice controlled, deep breathing as described in Chapter 5.
- Scan your body. Notice any areas that are tense and focus your attention on relaxing those muscles.
- Allow yourself to visualize a safe place of your choosing. This can be a place you have been to before, or one that you create in your mind, such as a beautiful beach, a lake, a special home, or a cozy room. Feel the ground underneath you or the softness of the chair you imagine sitting on. For some of you this may be a place that you hope to go to once you recover from surgery.
- Try to engage your senses by noticing the sights, the sounds, the sensations. Is there a cool breeze? Is the warm sun shining on your face? Stay in this place for a few minutes and just enjoy these sensations.
- Now visualize yourself healed from the surgery. Work on creating a positive image of your body feeling and functioning better. Picture yourself in your safe place feeling strong and well. You may see yourself there alone or with others. All that matters is that you just try to enjoy the experience of visualizing this positive surgical outcome.
- You may find using a mantra or chant helpful. Some possibilities include the following:

Breathe in strength, Breathe out fear,
May I be safe, May I be strong, May I be healthy,
I have everything that I need to heal.

- If you begin to have your worried thoughts, that's okay; just acknowledge them but then gently turn your attention back to your beautiful, healed outcome.
- Continue to breathe deeply and smoothly until you are ready to shift your attention back. Always remember the power and strength of your mind; remember that you can bring yourself back to a place of comfort, optimism, and strength anytime you need it.
- If practicing this in the hospital, you may want to bring your headset or AirPods and listen to some soothing music or a relaxation sound to help tune out the noise around you.

Post-Surgery Experience

After cardiac surgery you will usually be kept in a post-op room, where you will be closely monitored until your care team feel that you have stabilized and you are ready to be moved either to the intensive care unit (ICU) or cardiology ward, depending on what surgery you have undergone.

You have a right to privacy in the hospital just like you do in any other walk of life. Make sure that staff respect this right by using bed screens and giving you the opportunity to use bed baths or commodes in private. If you need help getting dressed, this should be done with discretion and respect.

You may find yourself attached to various types of medical equipment. It can be useful to understand what they are. If you would like to know more, you can ask your medical team what will be required for you so that you know what to expect.

Post-Surgery Recovery

Craig has always considered surgery to be like a marathon. He focuses all of his energy and determination on getting through the procedure and recovery, setting himself goals along the journey.

Focusing on recovery and the hope of getting better is what gets us through surgery and hospitalization. The length of time it takes to recover from surgery depends on the procedure involved, but some general points may help:

- Initially you will probably feel very groggy and sleepy. You may also feel some pain and possibly quite unwell. Taking things each moment at a time is effort enough.

- Ask for anything that might make you feel a bit more comfortable, for example an extra pillow, a fan, a cool compress on your forehead, some ice cubes on your lips, or help moving into a more comfortable position.
- If you don't feel up to visitors, then explain this to them and kindly ask them to come back later or the following day.
- Sleep is how the body recovers, but this is not always easy on a busy cardiac ward between beeping heart monitors, nurses' ongoing monitoring visits, doctors' rounds, and requests for ECGs and X-rays.

Meals are usually at set times, and you might be woken up for breakfast or for your bed to be changed. Try and work around this to get as much rest as you need while being assertive about how much disruption you can tolerate (e.g., if you don't want to be woken up for breakfast, ask for a note to be hung on your bed stating this).

- Once you start to feel a little better, it can help you to set goals. For example, eating your first food, being able to sit up in bed, getting to stand, and going for a little walk are all significant achievements.
- Remember there might be setbacks along the way and always pace yourself by listening to your body.
- Don't suffer in silence; report any unmanageable pain or discomfort. It is important to keep pain under control rather than letting it get really bad. In addition to pain medication, you can also use relaxation and meditation techniques to manage pain.
- Accept help. You have gotten through what most people have not, and the consequences of being born with a heart condition reach far beyond the physical symptoms.
- Plan treats for yourself and set goals for when you feel up to it.
- Before and after hospitalization it can help to prepare the body with healing techniques such as reiki, acupuncture, reflexology, or Indian head massage.

Longer–Term Recovery

- Eat well. Your body has been through an ordeal. It will take time to build yourself back up. It might help to take supplements or a tonic (as approved by your medical team).
- You will likely feel bruised and sore for some time after your procedure depending on how invasive it has been. Continue to take care of yourself and do lots of self-soothing activities such as keeping cozy,

spending time with loved ones, and watching or reading comforting books or films.

• It may be that you can now do more than you could before your hospital stay, or it might be that you cannot do as much. Either way requires an adjustment to how you see your body, especially if you are left with a new scar or have been fitted with a cardiac device such as a pacemaker. If you have any loss of functioning, it is okay to grieve and process this loss.

• Pace yourself. Of course, you want to get better and back to your "normal" self, but appreciate what you have been through and give yourself time to heal physically and emotionally.

Taking Medications

Part of managing your cardiac condition may involve taking a complicated cocktail of drugs. It is useful to keep a list of all of the medications and doses that you require so that you can readily share it with your healthcare providers and in event of an emergency. It is important to take your medications as prescribed and to report any side effects. Some individuals find that organizing their pills in a medication dispenser helps them to keep track of their correct dosages.

Coping during a Global Pandemic

The pandemic has been very difficult, because I don't look like there's anything wrong with me. When I attempt to advocate for myself at work, explaining that I'm high risk, I've been told by coworkers that I'm "being overly cautious." I have also had managers completely dismiss my concerns regarding COVID-19, ignoring my requests or suggestions for safety reasons, until I have a doctor's note that they can't ignore.

—Lenae, 33 years old, United States

It is perfectly natural to feel anxious about the COVID-19 pandemic, more so if you have an underlying health condition. At the start of the outbreak, some people with a CHC were advised by their healthcare providers that they were "extremely clinically vulnerable" to the COVID-19 virus (such as some individuals with Fontan circulation, cyanosis, pulmonary hypertension, heart failure, or immunocompromised)[18] and were advised to clinically shield (stay at home) during acute phases of the outbreak. As regulations have relaxed, many individuals have expressed confusion over the conflicting reports, advice, and questions about vaccine hesitancy. Having a trusted healthcare provider we can turn to for advice is essential during this trying time.

In reality, the COVID-19 outbreak has the potential to increase health inequalities impacting on those of us with an underlying health condition physically, financially, and socially. Studies have found increased risk to mental health of shielding and disruption to accessing cardiac care in the CHC population,[19] while media narratives about people with underlying health conditions can add to a sense of being marginalized and dispensable.[20]

As such, it is even more important to look after ourselves during these uncertain times. If you are feeling more stressed or anxious, it is important to recognize this as a normal response to an abnormal situation and draw on coping strategies to manage these feelings. Self-care, self-compassion, and finding ways to stay connected to others are all vital.

The good news is that one study found that while those of us with a CHC have found the pandemic challenging and it has made some of us more aware of our condition, we have also been able to draw on our lived experience of medical uncertainty to cope. Further, emotional regulation (see Chapter 6) is associated with increased posttraumatic growth during the outbreak.[21]

Some Tips for Coping

- Be proactive; follow guidance for your condition (from trusted sources).
- Share contact details of key healthcare providers and an action plan with loved ones in case you become unwell.
- Contact your healthcare providers for advice; don't sit on worries. Most healthcare providers offer telemedicine visits during acute phases of the pandemic, to allow for video contact with your doctor to minimize added viral exposure.
- Be sure to still contact healthcare providers for non-COVID-19 health worries.
- Remember it is normal to feel more anxious during abnormal times. Find a way to express how you are feeling, and draw on coping

techniques, such as grounding, breathing exercises, distraction, and practicing self-compassion (draw from Chapters 5–8).

- If there are things you can no longer do, make sure you substitute them with alternative enjoyable activities.
- Make sure you are finding ways to connect with others.
- Avoid overabsorbing news and negative messaging from the media and online.
- Avoid triggers of medical trauma (such as images of ventilators, etc.).
- Maintain self-care, structure, and routine and a healthy life balance.
- Communicate your needs with your employers and seek legal advice or support from advocacy organizations if you feel like you are being marginalized because of your condition or if you are experiencing financial hardship.
- Hospital visiting and being accompanied to appointments have been limited during the pandemic, challenging essential social support during these stressful times. If this is the case, check with your hospital to see if concessions can be made, given your long-term condition. If not, try to find other ways to keep in contact with loved ones (e.g., FaceTime).

Dealing with a Deterioration in Health

Dealing with a decline in your health or difficult medical news can naturally evoke a range of emotions such as anger, frustration, sadness, disappointment, and anxiety. These feelings are a perfectly normal response to disappointing news. You may have concerns about the impact of this on others, your finances, loss of independence, or facing further medical procedures. You may have to deal with a new set of symptoms, such as arrhythmia, or a new medicine regime. Finding ways to process your feelings and articulate your concerns is important and you can draw on the techniques described previously to process these feelings and communicate how you are feeling to others in your social network. There may be parts of this situation that you can't do anything about which can trigger a grieving process. In this case, it is completely understandable to feel sad, teary, and frustrated. In time, when you feel better able to accept these changes, it can be useful to reset your goals accordingly. It is important to make sure that you are still having enjoyable and rewarding experiences and a sense of purpose.

Living with Heart Failure

Receiving a diagnosis of heart failure can be scary, and you may have a lot of questions about how this may affect you in terms of your symptoms and treatment options. A heart failure diagnosis is made when your heart isn't functioning as well or pumping as strongly as it should. Some of the symptoms can include increased fatigue, water retention, shortness of breath, bloating, and weight gain. For some individuals, heart failure is a chronic condition. If your symptoms are managed, you may be able to live your life as you normally would, unless the deterioration in the function of your heart begins to progress. Depending upon where you live and your symptoms, your cardiologist may refer you to a heart failure specialist or, if you are at or near a large hospital, they may refer you to a heart failure center, which ideally would be integrated into your ACHD center.

Specialist Insights on Living with Heart Failure

Dr. Daniel Jacoby, MD, Associate Professor and Director of the Cardiomyopathy Program and the Comprehensive Heart Failure Program at Yale New Haven Hospital, describes heart failure, especially in the CHC community, as a very broad term, noting that most of the literature about diagnosis and treatment is focused on *traditional heart failure*, or those with acquired heart disease.[22] Dr. Jacoby notes that individuals generally fall into one of two categories, either chronic compensated heart failure or acute decompensated heart failure, as indicated by the ACC/AHA guidelines.

After receiving a diagnosis, depending on where the individual is are on this broad spectrum, the treatment recommendations may vary. There may be some individuals who fall into the chronic category who may be sent home with recommendations for medication, diet, or lifestyle changes. Others may require hospitalization to help get their symptoms under control.

Some of the current treatment options are as follows:

• Identification of the cause and attempt to address it (e.g., in the case of valve replacement)

- Medication
- A pacemaker (an implantable device which helps control your heart rhythm)
- An implantable cardioverter-defibrillator (ICD), which is implanted and able to perform cardioversion and/or pacing of the heart
- Cardiac resynchronization therapy (an implantable pacemaker which can coordinate the function of the left and right ventricles)
- Ventricular assist device (VAD) (an implanted device which assists in cardiac circulation and pumps blood)
- Heart transplant

Coping with Heart Failure at Home

During this time self-care is a must. Having an understanding of why you are prescribed a medication or other treatment recommendation is important. You may be asked to weigh yourself frequently and keep a record of your symptoms, fluid intake, and weight. This information can help determine if you are retaining fluids and if you may need a change in your treatment regime.

Your lifestyle may need to shift after this diagnosis. Generally, individuals are instructed to reduce their salt intake, cut back on alcohol, and stop smoking. Your doctor may recommend that if your symptoms allow, you stay physically active. If you are employed, you may or may not need to reduce the number of hours you work, or if your job involves heavy lifting, you may need to speak with your supervisor about shifting to a less strenuous job. Since this isn't always possible, this can be very hard for many because it can affect them financially. Some individuals decide to leave their jobs and, with their doctor's help, can apply for disability benefits. By working together with your specialized care team, you can come up with a treatment plan to try to manage your symptoms and prevent your condition from getting worse.

Because of our long history of living with a CHC, many of us had been told by our doctors that we would be unable to do certain things in our life and often we ended up being able to do these things. There are some of us who may have been given a poor prognosis years ago, but decades on we are still living our lives. Consider the child who is told they may not live past the age of 13, but who is now 30 years old. Consider the teen who is told they shouldn't exercise but then ends up exercising regularly, without any problem, and frequently jogs in many 5K races. It is understandable, then, for those individuals who are referred for a heart transplant workup, that these experiences can sometimes feed into an overall sense of doubt or denial. They may feel that they were given inaccurate information in the past or that they "beat their CHC" before, and this overall belief could play into not believing or taking the recommendation seriously. However, to ensure the best outcome following a diagnosis of heart failure, it is vital that lifestyle recommendations are taken seriously.

Dr. Jacoby explains that, if required, the earlier a referral is made to the transplant team, the more prepared the team can be, which will enable them to give us the best chance for a positive outcome. Often individuals with a CHC are referred too late, which increases the chances of not being cleared to have the transplant. This could be due to a number of issues, including, but not limited to, poor kidney function, high pressure in the lungs, or substance abuse. Although the topic of conversation was a very serious one, Dr. Jacoby ended our discussion with this hopeful message: "We can handle just about anything, but we need the proper time and preparation."

To that end, Dr. Jacoby recommends that if you have a moderate or complex CHC you begin having a conversation with your cardiologist about your risks for heart failure and the possible need for future transplant. Often, this isn't a topic that healthcare providers like to talk about, but he believes that not knowing is actually doing us more harm than good. While having this conversation, many of us will be told that a transplant is not likely to be in our future, but others may be told it is something that will need to be revisited every year, or every few years.

Preparing for Transplant

I want to know so badly what it feels like to walk, ride a horse, swim, and run with a two-chambered heart. I sometimes think about my life post-transplant and, quite honestly, dream about what not being out of breath from normal activities will feel like.

—Lauren, 27 years old, United States

Once referred for a transplant, individuals may require hospitalization to manage their symptoms. Heart transplants are not suited for all patients, so there will be a lot of testing required to help the team determine if you would be a suitable candidate. This will require a lot of testing, interviewing, and paperwork (for consent; and in countries with private healthcare, for insurance approval). If it is found that the center is unable to take you on as a transplant patient, they can sometimes refer you to a center which is more experienced or equipped to deal with your individual needs. Some individuals may find that there are some additional medical issues which deem them unsuitable (such as kidney function or high pressure in the lungs). In this case, some may be given the option for a ventricular assist device (VAD), a mechanical pump used to assist the heart's pumping mechanism, which may or may not help to improve those issues so that you may qualify for a transplant in the future.

If you are deemed to be a candidate, most individuals are hospitalized and can face a waiting process. Dawn Lorentson, LCSW at Yale New Haven Hospital's Adult Congenital Heart Disease Center,[23] notes that this can be very difficult, even more so during the COVID-19 pandemic, which has restricted individuals from having visitors. She suggests that one of the best things a person in this situation can do is to try to find ways to assert some control. This may include setting up your room with objects that bring you joy and comfort, having your partner or spouse cuddle with you when visiting, or encouraging visits from family and friends (if the hospital allows; if not, having plenty of FaceTime, phone calls, and messaging with them). Scheduling time to speak with a therapist, clergy, or connecting with a peer mentor who has been through a transplant can also help. Finding things to occupy your time is also important; some examples include puzzles, art, letter writing, and/or a good TV Box-set. Drawing from the tools and techniques described through Chapters 5–9 to help with self-care, sleep, managing overwhelming feelings, and distraction should help. You may also benefit from the *Visualizing Your Recovery* exercise described earlier in this chapter, focusing on life after a transplant.

Ms. Lorenston explained that it is important to try to talk about the very conflicted feelings around waiting for your new heart. She also suggested working on *meaning-making* with a supportive friend, family member, or therapist. This involves processing and coming to terms with questions such as *What are my priorities in life? What is important to me?* and *How can I communicate it with those I care about?* Processing possible feelings of remorse and grief for the donor and their family members also can come up at this time. Preparing for post-transplant life is another important task that she recommends individuals focus on while they are waiting. Some individuals find that working through these complex issues with a therapist can be beneficial.

Although I was born with a heart defect, never once did I think I'd ever need or get a heart transplant. Well, that time came and the news was hard to accept. The thought of a heart transplant was very overwhelming, but deep down I knew it was something I had to accept. The transplant was not easy, but in the end worth it. I'm 3 years post transplant and I feel great! My quality of life has improved so much that even 3 years later I'm surprised at what I can now do!

—*Charlotte, 58 years old, United States*

Managing Chronic Symptoms: Pacing, Prioritizing, and Planning

Studies indicate that people with a CHC are more likely to experience chronic symptoms, including pain,[24] fatigue, and breathlessness, which can have a negative impact on quality of life. The toll of living with these chronic symptoms on our mental health, well-being, and daily functioning can be enormous, especially when they are deemed "unexplained." Often these "nonacute" and "hidden" symptoms are poorly acknowledged or addressed by healthcare systems and may even be invalidated with remarks such as *"You shouldn't be feeling this way"* or *"No one else with your condition reports this,"* which can add to the burden of trying to manage them.

Unexplained chest pain has caused considerable anguish over the years. Although these episodes happen rarely, they have often been serious enough to present to the hospital emergency department. In most cases they have resulted in being discharged without any conclusive explanation for chest pain and symptoms experienced. How about: It is quite frustrating when symptoms and concerns are not understood or explained by medical professionals.. Whilst medical professionals are often able to rule things out, not being able to diagnose or explain what is happening does not alleviate any of the concerns or the reasons for presenting to the emergency department in the first place.

—*Benjamin, 39 years old, Australia*

Chronic symptoms can also receive less support from our loved ones, peers, educators, and colleagues, attracting, comments such as *"But you look so well"* or *"I get tired, too."* It is one thing to support someone through an obvious, time-limited, medical crisis such as cardiac surgery. It is quite another being there for them for months or years as they manage a daily battle with chronic symptoms. For example, colleagues don't witness that as a result of turning up and giving your all at work you may have to rest the next day, or friends seldom grasp that after attending a wedding you may spend the weekend in your pajamas. As a result, you may feel more isolated in dealing with these symptoms. Even others with a CHC who do not suffer from chronic symptoms can find it hard to understand. Finding ways to manage these symptoms while communicating the impact they have on you is essential to psychological well-being.

Chronic symptoms can lead you to feeling frustrated with, and fighting against, your body. This can result in self-criticism, body image issues, pushing yourself relentlessly, and even self-punitive behaviors, all of which can end up making your symptoms worse and impacting negatively on your sense of self and mood. You may feel there is little point in following a healthy diet or trying to exercise if you are just going to feel bad anyway. It is important to recognize that your body is doing the best it can for you. You may want to refer to the section in Chapter 8 on "Relationship with Yourself" if this is an issue for you. Recognizing your limits and looking after yourself are key to being your best self.

The three Ps—Pacing, Prioritizing, and Planning—are useful for self-management of these chronic symptoms (see Figure 9.3). Often when we feel a bit better, we overdo it. Or we might push ourselves through the tiredness or pain and suffer for it the next day or even week, known as "boom and bust." In reality, to gain control of these symptoms and function optimally, it is important to start listening to your body and recognizing your own limits.

It can help to think about yourself as a container that has most of your energy at the start of each day (or whenever the best time of day is for you). You don't want to end up using your energy up too fast, which would leave you depleted by the end of the day. Often when that happens, we end up paying for it later, often waking up the next day with less vigor and motivation than usual. Using your energy wisely throughout the day rather than using it all up at once will help you sustain it and make the most out of your days. Ideally you will pace yourself so that you have a little left by the end of your day. Occasionally you might need to borrow energy from the next day, for example to attend a special event such as a wedding. If this is the case, and you come home depleted, then you can plan a "rest day" afterward to compensate.

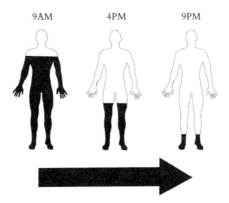

Pacing Planning Prioritizing

Figure 9.3 Pacing yourself.

Some people with chronic symptoms find it useful to split the day up into three parts (morning, afternoon, and evening), only making commitments in two of the parts, allowing themselves to rest and recover for the other third. It is also okay to prioritize what matters to you rather than "wasting" your precious resources on things that are less important to you. It can be hard to say no, and you may want to refer to the section on "Assertive Communication" in Chapter 8 to explore how to set boundaries further. Being able to effectively communicate what it means for you to pace yourself and manage your symptoms to others is important.

You may also find it useful to use labor-saving devices, take frequent micro-breaks, and if required use disability access (for example, to avoid a flight of stairs, steep climb, or far walk from a parking spot). If possible, working part time or finding a way to work for yourself where you can better manage your own work schedule can also make a huge difference.

Palliative Care

Palliative care is a type of healthcare or resource for individuals with a serious illness. It can be accessed at any stage of illness and is different from a hospice, as it is not just for end-of-life care. It can be helpful to anyone who is suffering from a disability or suffering in relation to their medical condition. Unlike a hospice, patients can continue to receive their curative treatments while receiving palliative care, which focuses on helping individuals manage their symptoms, discomfort, and improve their quality of life.

Some of the services which can be provided include pain management, the planning and coordination of care, and mental health treatment. In the United States, insurance providers may cover many of these services. Your ACHD specialist may be able to refer you to a palliative care team; usually these services are based in a hospital, outpatient setting, or long-term care facility.

10

Taking the Wheel

In times of crisis, people reach for meaning. Meaning is our strength. Our survival may depend on seeking and finding it.

—Viktor Frankl[1]

Ultimately, it is healthiest to focus on what you *can* do, as opposed to what you can't do, and to define yourselves beyond any health struggles. The better we are able to manage the physical and psychological challenges of our congenital heart conditions (CHCs), the more we can embrace the other parts of ourselves and live as fully as possible. In taking control of your condition, it is important to give yourself time and space to process your experiences and feelings while searching for healthy meaning and purpose. Further, when you retrieve your power, emotional healing can occur.

Colette is a 34-year-old woman with a complex CHC. Despite having several surgeries and a bout of endocarditis, she was able to get through college and graduate school. She is now working in her field of choice as a guidance counselor and mentor to high school students. In her spare time she volunteers at a camp for children with CHCs, and she enjoys traveling to places where she can enjoy the warm water.

Congenital Heart Condition: A "Hidden" Disability and Disability Pride

My north star growing up was to live a normal life. It was a time when having a birth defect seemed to somehow make you the subject of pity or less of a person. Not wanting that and since I could disguise most of my limitations fairly well, I was determined that only my family and close friends would be told I had CHD. While

now it is much easier to tell someone, it still gives me a sense of pride when someone I
tell says, "I never knew you had CHD." In retrospect, I'm not sure that all the time
and energy I put into covering my CHD did me any real good.

—Mitch, 59 years old, United States

Disability is defined as "a physical or mental impairment that has a 'sub-stantial' and 'long-term' negative effect on your ability to do normal daily activities."[2] Some people with a CHC self-identify as having a disability while others don't, and the nature of living with a CHC can make this challenging to define. For many, daily functioning is close to normal, yet life can be punctuated by periods of sudden, acute illness that can result in serious medical interventions such as open heart surgery, device implant, or hospitalization to control an arrhythmia. For some, these acute episodes may result in a temporary or permanent inability to work and the need to apply for financial assistance from the government, assistance with mo-bility, or disability access. Such repeated interruptions can negatively im-pact your overall health, well-being, confidence, education, and career. In this situation, it can be difficult to establish how much your health impacts your "daily functioning" even following "recovery" from a more acute episode.

Some people choose not to identify as having a disability because they worry about being "reduced to their condition" and facing discrimination. Identifying as having a disability may be associated with being stigmatized, feeling different, and social exclusion. Arguably, this is "internalized dis-crimination," but often this is based on very real experiences at work or socially after sharing information about their condition. Others may not identify with the term because they don't believe that their normal daily life is impacted enough, or they don't want to accept assistance that they may not need. Revealing your condition and risking the consequences may seem like a battle too many, while keeping this part of you hidden can negatively impact on self-esteem and mean that you are unable to access the support and resources you have a right to. "*Who should I tell about my condi-tion and when should I tell them?*" is a dilemma many of us have experienced throughout our lives.

The reality is that disability is a common experience, with over 1 billion people or about 15% of the global population currently experiencing dis-ability.[3] While some people worry that being labeled as "disabled" means they have "given up," in reality a growing body of evidence suggests that embracing your condition and being proud of your ability to manage it is more empowering than "rejecting" this part of you.[4] The "disability pride" social movement recognizes that living with a serious health condition can impact our sense of self, rights, and access to society's resources.

Often people with a disability are marginalized, finding it harder to access the rights, responsibilities, roles, resources, and relationships that society offers. These five Rs[5] are usually obtainable through public and social institutions and local communities (e.g., schools, colleges, health services, and employers) yet can be "just out of reach" when they are designed for the healthy majority. Research has found that those of us living with a serious lifelong health condition can share a number of disadvantages with other minority groups, including disparities in civil rights, discrimination, income, education, employment, and underrepresentation in the media and politics (when was the last time you saw someone with a CHC being accurately represented in a Hollywood film, soap opera, or novel?),[6] imposing unnecessary daily barriers to normal life.

Social models of disability aim to challenge discrimination by using the word "impairment" to describe the actual attributes (or lack of attributes) that affect a person (such as an inability to walk or breathe independently) whereas the word "disability" is used to refer to the restrictions caused by society when it does not give equivalent attention and accommodation to the needs of individuals with impairments.[7]

Ableism, the assumption that we need to be "fixed" while treating able-bodied people as the norm, leads to a society organized to accommodate the majority (for example, an expectation to be able to work 9 to 5, full-time). More often than not we don't recognize these barriers because we have grown up in a world where this is the norm. Yet they can add to the daily burden of living with a serious lifelong health condition beyond the direct impact on us physically. As a result, we may wonder why we find everything such a struggle when our peers do not, resulting in self-blame and even low mood. By recognizing these invisible barriers we can make sense of our lived experience and empower ourselves by understanding our rights.

Often, to access disability rights, for example in the workplace and education sector, or to access financial assistance, it is necessary to tick that "disability" box. "Owning" your condition, being aware of your rights, and proactively seeking meaningful roles, your own community, and places to belong (such as through CHC support groups) may be necessary to better get your needs met. It may also be beneficial to seek support through advocacy if you find that you are being marginalized or you are unable to access resources (such as health and life insurance and other employer based benefits). For example, if your employer discriminated against you and as a result, you are faced with "constructive dismissal", which leaves you with little choice but to resign.

It is important to recognize that everyone with a disability is different and with a wide spectrum of identities and privilege. This intersectionality can in part explain why one person with a certain condition can function better than someone else. For example, someone who has a CHC and is also struggling financially may have difficulty accessing the healthcare they need.[8]

Many people have fought long and hard to establish awareness, rights, and equality for people who are disadvantaged by a disability, for example in the United Nations Convention on the Rights of Persons with Disabilities (UN-CRPD) discussed later in this chapter. The disability pride movement aims to create a counterculture that values diversity while challenging systemic ableism. This is something you may choose to engage with.

How you term your condition is a very personal issue, and you need to do what works for and empowers you. It may be that you use different terms in different situations, guided by your own wisdom, judgment, and lived experience. What matters most is that you are in control, that you feel only pride in how you choose to manage your condition, and that you are self-compassionate about any additional barriers you face.

Know Your Rights

Speaking of rights, it is useful to know what they are. The Human Rights Act (1998) in the United Kingdom outlines the basic rights and freedoms that belong to everyone in the world and that must be followed by healthcare providers, educators, and employers. Under the Human Rights Act, "disability" is a "protected characteristic," which means it is against the law to discriminate against anyone on the basis of their disability. Further, many countries have adopted specific "patient rights," which are embedded within healthcare legislation.

Patient Rights

- The right to access health services
- The right to access good quality of care
- The right to receive treatment from appropriately qualified and experienced staff
- The right to be involved in making decisions about your medications and treatments
- The right to be protected from abuse and neglect
- The right to be treated by all staff with respect and confidentiality
- The right to access your medical records
- The right to informed consent
- The right to complain if you aren't happy or if things go wrong
- The right to make decisions about end-of-life care

United Nations Convention on the Rights of Persons with Disabilities

The United Nations Convention on the Rights of Persons with Disabilities (UN-CRPD) is an international human rights treaty intended to protect the rights and dignity of people with a disability, first adopted by the United Nations General Assembly in 2006. As of July 2020, it has 163 signatories and 182 parties, 181 states, and the European Union. Parties to the UN-CRPD are required to promote and protect the human rights of anyone with a disability who is entitled to equality by law.[9]

The eight guiding principles underlying the UN-CRPD are as follows:

1. Respect for inherent dignity, individual autonomy (including the freedom to make one's own choices), and independence of persons
2. Nondiscrimination
3. Full and effective participation and inclusion in society
4. Respect for difference and acceptance of persons with disabilities as part of human diversity and humanity
5. Equality of opportunity
6. Accessibility
7. Equality between men and women
8. Respect for the evolving capacities of children with disabilities and respect for the right of children with disabilities to preserve their identities

Further, in the United States, the Americans with Disabilities Act (1990)[10] prohibits discrimination against individuals with disabilities in all areas of public life, including jobs, schools, transportation, and all public and private areas that are open to the general public.

Navigating the World of Education and Work

When my heart started to palpitate in 2013, due to stress and anxiety, my manager underestimated the difficulties I was facing and compared it to short-term stress that a member of her family had experienced. This meant that I wasn't given the support that I needed.

—Zeb, 55 years old, United Kingdom

Many people with a CHC are able to study full time and work the usual 9–5 schedule without any issues while some individuals may struggle with a "normal" full-time work or study pattern. Others may find this temporarily challenging following a period of ill health or surgery. It is important to find a study/work-health-life balance that works for you, which may change over time. For some, traditional studying/working patterns may not be ideally suited. Times are changing, and there are more opportunities these days to accommodate flexible work patterns, working from home, and hybrid work patterns.

A range of studies have demonstrated a negative impact of CHD on both educational attainment and employment status.[11] Report that compared to healthy adults, even among the healthiest adults with CHD, there are significant decrements in both employment and lifetime earnings.[12] As such, it is important to be aware of your educational and employment rights.[13] It is important to inform your place of education or employment about your health condition because if your health impacts your daily functioning you should be entitled to "reasonable adjustments" to your study pattern or workplace duties.

Unfortunately, some people with a CHC report facing discrimination in their education or workplace. Discrimination is defined as being disadvantaged for a reason that relates to your disability, and it may be direct (e.g., missing out on a promotion), indirect (e.g., a rule or policy which has a worse impact on someone with a protected characteristic), harassment (being treated in a way that violates your dignity), or victimization.[14]

Often it is subtle, perhaps unintentional but damaging nonetheless, especially when you are exposed to it repeatedly. Workplace bullying is a risk factor for disability retirement.[15] Discrimination is illegal, unacceptable, and should be reported.

If you are experiencing discrimination at work or in education, make sure you are keeping a record of what is going on that so that you can report your experience to Human Resources. It is also helpful to join a union if you have one, and you can also seek advocacy and legal advice and draw on legislation relevant to where you live (e.g., the Americans with Disabilities Act).

Some people with a CHC debate about whether to tell prospective employers about their condition. Depending on which country you live in, it may be necessary to tell your employers about your condition to be protected legally. While disability law should protect us from discrimination, the reality is that it can be hard to prove you have not been selected at interview or subject to constructive dismissal because of your condition. In the United Kingdom, there are disability employment advisors in every job center. They can also advise about work-related benefits. Universities and colleges also have disability services that can offer support and advice.

If your health condition is such that you are unable to work, then you should be able to claim disability payments. If you are unable to work due to your health condition, it is likely that you will need to go through an assessment process to access any financial assistance. This process will vary depending on where you live. It can be arduous and you may be able to access advocacy and advice from a CHC support organization or similar. It is still important to have goals and a sense of purpose even if you aren't working.

It can be hard to battle this kind of treatment when you have already had to fight so much,[16] but don't let anyone make you feel like you are less deserving of a career or education because of your condition. You are just as entitled as anyone else. It may well be that you need to find your own way to fulfill your goals and ambitions. Some people with a CHC report factoring their condition into the choices they make about what to study or which jobs to go for, particularly if their condition impacts on their health daily (for example, fatigue).

Despite having a CHC, and being in and out of hospital since infancy, Susan worked hard to gain her professional training. She was delighted to get a job with an

*understanding team leader. He let her manage her workload by adjusting her respon-
sibilities to accommodate her condition while still fulfilling the needs of the role. When
she returned to work following another cardiac surgery, he encouraged her, helping her
work to her strengths and getting her more paid hours, which helped to build her confidence. However, when he was promoted, his replacement took issue with Susan getting
"special treatment." She raised her work plan during a team meeting, in front of her
colleagues, suggesting Susan should take on more to fulfill her contracted hours and job
description. Susan was blindsided and felt shamed just like she had been by mean kids
during childhood who picked on her for "using" her condition to "get out of" gym class
despite "looking well." She tried to advocate for herself, but this just led to strained relationships and when pressure continued she found little support. She didn't have the
energy to raise it formally. Instead, she decided to leave her post and found a way to
work for herself where she could manage her own workload.*

Seeking Therapy

> *I never thought much about seeking mental health support. When I mentioned my
> pre-surgery anxiety to my primary care doctor, she suggested I see a therapist. It was
> the best thing I ever did. She helped me mentally prepare for my surgery and gave me
> tools to cope with my anxiety.*
>
> —Lee, 64 years old, United States

In Chapter 2 we talked about how the majority of us in need of mental
health support are not receiving it, yet receiving mental health treatment
can actually improve our heart health. So why are so few individuals accessing therapy? From our experience working with many individuals with
CHC, we have listed some of the obstacles.

Stigma: Unfortunately there continues to be stigma attached to mental
health treatment which can be influenced by culture, family beliefs, or society. Some people experience feelings of shame or embarrassment about
their emotional challenges. Some people have even been told that they
should "be able to deal with it," "be strong and work it out on their own."
Others report feeling reluctant to admit they are struggling emotionally because they do not want to upset their loved ones or caregivers. In reality, it
takes a lot of courage and strength to be honest with ourselves about what
feelings and/or issues are troubling us, and even more to reach out and ask
for help.

Poor or no insurance coverage: Attending therapy can be a commitment,
both of time and of finances. In the United States some people experience

difficulty locating a mental health provider who is willing to accept their insurance. If paying out of pocket, the fees can be high, which for many can be a huge barrier to treatment.

A lack of appropriate mental health care providers: This will vary based on where you are living. If you are being cared for by an accredited adult congenital heart disease (ACHD) center in the United States, or an ACHD specialized center in other countries such as the United Kingdom, there should be a mental health provider as part of their team. People living in more rural areas can find it more challenging to access therapy locally, especially with specialist CHC expertise. Fortunately, since the COVID-19 pandemic, accessing therapy in some states in the United States has become easier due to emergency orders and telehealth coverage mandates, which require commercial health plans and Medicaid to cover these services. Further, teletherapy has become more accessible and standard in most countries around the world.

Long waiting lists: For countries with public healthcare, such as the United Kingdom, waiting lists to access local psychology teams can be very long while few specialist centers have psychologists embedded in their team. Accessing therapy privately is costly, with few people having private health coverage.

Tips for Finding a Therapist

Finding a good therapist isn't always easy. It requires research, time, and motivation. The best person to ask is generally your primary care physician or cardiologist, who can make a referral to a psychologist or mental health specialist. Some primary care offices and ACHD centers have a mental health professional as part of their team. If that is not the case, word of mouth might be the best bet. If you are comfortable, ask your friends and family if they can recommend anyone. Getting a personal recommendation gives you the opportunity to get a referral from someone you trust.

As an alternative, in the United States, your insurance company should be able to send you a list of their in-network providers in your area. Other referral sources include local religious institutions, psychological training institutes, counseling centers, and websites such as *Psychology Today* (United States).

Most countries have professional organizations which list licensed practitioners such as the American Psychological Association (APA) in the
United States and the British Psychological Society (BPS) or the Health
and Social Care Professions Council (HCPC), which regulate healthcare
professionals across the United Kingdom. Therapy is typically done by a
number of different healthcare professionals, including psychologists, clinical social workers, psychiatrists, and marriage and family therapists, in the
United States.

Once you have a few names, it is best to try to speak with two or three
different therapists to get a sense of their style, experience, areas of interest,
and price point. Feeling safe and comfortable with the individual you
choose is very important. Some of the questions to ask include the following: How long have you been practicing? Do you have any experience
working with a CHC patient, or other serious chronic illness? What are the
modalities you frequently use? In the United States you may also call the
state licensing board to ensure their license is in good standing. If you do
not have or want to use your private insurance, you will then need to pay
the therapist directly. If this is the case, sometimes therapists will slide their
fee scale if you don't have any insurance reimbursement (United States).
This is a conversation that is best to have before you begin therapy with
that individual. Another option is to contact a local university, professional
training institution, or local clinic. Often these organizations can help to
locate an experienced provider. Finally, you can always contact free hotlines
for crisis support. We have listed a few numbers in the Appendix.

What Type of Therapy?

Cognitive behavioral therapy (CBT) is the recommended and evidence-
based treatment for most anxiety disorders, including generalized anxiety
disorder, phobias, health anxiety, and panic disorder. CBT is also recommended for depression. Trauma-informed CBT, body psychotherapy, and
eye movement desensitization and reprocessing (EMDR)[17] have also been
recommended for medically related trauma disorders. Acceptance and commitment therapy (ACT) can be useful for helping you manage a long-term
health condition, while body psychotherapy is beneficial for people who
have experienced body trauma. Different approaches work for different

people, while the relationship with your therapist is just as important as the therapeutic modality. It is important to find someone with whom you feel safe, comfortable, and able to work.

Medication

Some people also find that antidepressant medication is useful for managing symptoms when your toolbox and/or therapy isn't helpful in reducing these uncomfortable feelings. This may be true during an acute crisis or particularly stressful time, or for more chronic or long-term symptoms. Whenever possible, we recommend adding therapy to your treatment regime if you are taking a psychotropic medication. The combination of the two treatment modalities has a much higher likelihood of reaching a full recovery.

It can sometimes be helpful to ask for medication, such as a tranquilizer, to help you sleep the night before a surgery or to calm your anxiety leading up to the day. Sometimes your specialist healthcare team can prescribe this medication for you. If that is not possible, they may be able to refer you to another physician who is seasoned in conducting a medication evaluation, such as a psychiatrist or advanced practice nurse practitioner.

It is always best for your congenital heart specialist to work together with other professionals whenever possible to explore what is the safest and best approach for you. It is important to always keep them in the loop about how you are feeling. Remember, you are the most important part of your treatment team in ensuring that you are receiving the care you need.

Genetic Counseling and Pregnancy Planning

I wish that I had known more about the genetic causes of CHC and the ongoing research involved. Although I had a CHC, I had no reason to think that I had Noonan's syndrome (NS) and that there was a 50% chance of me passing NS and CHC on to my child. It wasn't until after my son was diagnosed with NS that doctors even considered testing me. Having this knowledge before having my son would have better prepared me for his journey with CHC as well as helped me accept this new aspect of my identity.

—Molly, 37 years old, United States

Deciding whether or not to have children is something that requires more consideration for many individuals with a CHC. Most women with a CHC will cope well with pregnancy. There can be increased risks to you and the baby, and it is important to discuss this with your ACHD specialized care team if you are planning a pregnancy. You and your partner may be referred to a genetic counselor to get information on the likelihood of having a child with a CHC. Your ACHD specialist will most likely be able to refer you to someone who is knowledgeable in the field of genetics and congenital heart disease. This is known as pre-conception counseling. Pregnancy does place extra demand on the heart, and certain factors can increase risk in pregnancy for people with a CHC.[18] Some of the risk factors are listed next.

Risk Factors for Pregnancy

- Your ventricular (pump) function
- Any leaky or thickened heart valves or having a mechanical heart valve
- Your oxygen levels
- If you have pulmonary hypertension (high blood pressure in the blood vessels that supply the lungs)
- Any current or past heart rhythm problems
- Your symptoms before pregnancy
- Medication you are taking
- Other medical conditions and lifestyle factors, such as smoking

I was always told as a kid that I could do whatever I wanted, but when I transitioned into ACHD, suddenly there was all this new information that made me think about my future differently. Suddenly I was told that having a pregnancy would be high-risk and could possibly lower my life expectancy. That was a huge blow to me. I had never been told that growing up! My mom would ask at every heart appointment if I could "have a family someday," and the answer was always yes. Now all of a sudden the answer was very different.

—*Lenae, 33 years old, United States*

After meeting with your ACHD specialist, they may decide to arrange some additional testing or interventions in order to evaluate your current cardiac status. This will help them to get a good sense of the risks involved. This process can be a stressful time for many people, and deciding to go through a pregnancy is a personal decision. During this pregnancy evaluation, it is important that you do not stop any medication without consulting a medical professional. While there are many women who are able to carry a pregnancy safely, there are others for whom it is not recommended

During this evaluation process, it is important that you take care of yourself and try to keep your stress levels low. It is also important that you and your partner communicate your feelings about the possible risks and other options you may have. It can be helpful to invite them to accompany you during your doctor's appointments so they are aware of the full picture so that you can make the decision together.

There are other important aspects that are worth considering beyond physical risk. Some people worry about whether they have enough energy to raise young children. Others are concerned about their life expectancy or the impact of their health condition on their prospective family. These are clearly important issues that need to be carefully considered and discussed with your partner and wider social network. This may also influence if and when you decide to start a family. Some people with a CHC decide to start their family at a younger age than they may have otherwise or have a smaller family than they may have liked. Of course, no one can predict how things will go, but these are issues that are important to discuss with your care team and support network.

If your team agrees that it would be reasonable for you to try to become pregnant, it may be recommended that you are followed by a high-risk obstetrician or perinatologist. Pregnancy and delivery create many cardiovascular changes, as your heart must work a lot harder, which may put you and the baby at higher risk. In an ideal situation your ACHD team will work together with this provider through your pregnancy and birth. Your delivery plan may include recommendations for pain management, medication changes, and type of delivery (unplanned vaginal, induced, or cesarean delivery), and they may want to schedule the delivery so that a member of the cardiology team can be present. Your doctors may want to schedule some additional testing during your pregnancy, such as a fetal echocardiogram. It is important to remember that this evaluation process should be followed before each and every pregnancy. Even if you had a successful pregnancy once, it does not guarantee that your cardiac status will be the same for a second one.

There is a big difference between a pregnancy being high risk versus life threatening. For those who are advised against becoming pregnant, it is generally because the risks to you and the baby would be unacceptable and could likely be life threatening. Understandably, this news can be very difficult to hear. This recommendation is generally not something doctors take lightly; however, some women do decide to see another ACHD specialist for a second opinion. If the consensus is the same, understandably this is a loss that will need to be processed as a woman, and as a couple. Finding out that you are unable to have a baby because of the risks involved can be devastating and may trigger a type of grief or loss. It is important that you are supported during this time. We have some information on this in Chapter 4.

It is important to know that there are many women who have gone through this process and because of the possible risks involved have decided not to go forward with a pregnancy. Some decide to live their lives without having a child, and they enjoy the many other aspects such as their work, relationships, being a supportive aunt, loving their pets, and having freedom. Others may decide to pursue a child of their own through adoption or surrogacy. Deciding whether or not to have a child is a personal decision. There really is no right or wrong answer. What is important is that you make your decision in an informed and thoughtful way.

Ida is a 26-year-old woman who was recently told by her ACHD specialist that becoming pregnant was not recommended due to the many risks involved. She had always wanted to have a child and was understandably devastated. She initially considered taking the risk without her doctor's blessing; however, after taking some time and speaking with her family, she realized that having a baby that she may not be around to care for was not what she wanted. With the help of a counselor, she and her husband decided to adopt and now have a beautiful daughter whom she adores. Ida has been well enough to care for her little girl and enjoys watching her grow.

Creating a family—from a man's perspective: What is normal? Normal is what you make of your life, accepting everything that is thrown at you. Dealing with it to the best of your ability. This was the approach I took, when starting a family. I was 32. I was a Dad. I was in love with a baby! Did my CHC define decisions I made to become a father? No, it didn't, but it did make me more circumspect. I spoke to my cardiologist before we started trying for a baby, and once pregnant, we had in-depth heart scans to ensure our baby was not carrying a CHC. Choosing to start a family is a big decision with lifelong consequences. Congenital heart disease should not stand in the way, but I know it can, for many men. The only thing I would change if I had my time over again would be the chance to talk with other CHD men that were already fathers.

—Stuart, 55 years old, New Zealand

If you do have a baby, it is important to get all of the support you need. We address parenting issues in Chapter 8.

Getting Older

When I was born in 1958, my parents were told to go home and get pregnant again as I wouldn't survive long. But because of the incredible lifelong care I have received, especially by those trained in adults with CHD, I am still here and lead a pretty normal life despite my CHC and implanted ICD (implantable cardioverter-defibrillator). My husband and I will celebrate our 39th anniversary next year and have been blessed with two biological children and two grandchildren that we couldn't love more. Life is very, very good!

—Millie, 63 years old, United States

Growing older comes with mixed feelings for many. Some people worry about the loss of youth, change in appearance, and the increased risk of developing illness and cognitive decline. Rapidly changing technology has made it possible for many individuals with CHC to enter middle and even late age. For many with CHC, we welcome growing older, especially if we were given a shortened life expectancy in the past. This is a wonderful gift. There are many individuals with CHC who are able to experience graying hair and who enjoy their grandchildren and retirement. In many ways, we perhaps embrace aging with an enhanced sense of gratitude compared with our heart-healthy peers because we do not take it for granted.

Having CHC does not preclude us from developing other acquired illnesses. As we age, our risk factors for other illnesses increase as they do for our heart-healthy peers. In fact, some of the childhood medical treatments for CHC can put us at higher risk of complications later in life, so being followed by an ACHD specialist continues to be essential. Therefore, it is important to pay attention to our overall heart health by managing our weight, blood pressure, cholesterol, and sugar levels, and managing risk factors such as sedentary lifestyle, smoking, vaping, and substance use. Regular recommended screenings such as lipid checks, colonoscopy, cancer screening skin checks, thyroid exams, prostate exams for men, and mammograms and pelvic exams for women should also be scheduled, as they are for our heart-healthy peers. It is also important that you inform any new physician of your CHC as there may be medications or treatments which are contraindicated.

While there seems to be ample information on pregnancy and CHC, there is unfortunately very little information on perimenopause and menopause for this population. Once again, pioneering CHC-ers are paving the way, creating learning as we go. Menopause is a natural biological process which marks the end of a woman's menstrual cycle, and perimenopause is the transition time leading up to it. As more women with CHC are now entering middle (and late) age, this information will become increasingly important to them not only for health education but also for symptom management, if needed. Menopausal symptoms can include (but are not limited to) hot flashes, night sweats, mood changes, irregular periods, weight gain, and vaginal dryness. While hormone replacement therapy (HRT) is an option to help ease these symptoms for many, it does come with the increased risk of blood clots.[19]

Erectile dysfunction can be a concern for men. It can result as a side effect of medication or aging, or it can be rooted in psychological concerns around body image, intimacy, and trust. Again, it is important to discuss these concerns with your healthcare provider because sexual health is an important part of life and relationships. While it can feel difficult to raise these issues, your healthcare team will be used to discussing them.

> I remember in the 1960s when I was a teenager lying in bed at night, I wondered if I would still be alive in the year 2000. And now, thanks to the advances in medicine, the skill of the various surgeons who repaired me during my four open heart surgeries and the knowledge of the various cardiologists that have treated me over the years; here I am in my mid-seventies in 2021, enjoying my retirement!
>
> —Len James, 74 years old, United States

Advance Care Planning

Advance care planning is your opportunity to make decisions about the treatment you would want to receive at a time if and when you are unable to speak for yourself. It is a written statement of what type of medical care you want at the end of life. The paperwork involved will vary depending on where you live, and it is worthwhile exploring this with your healthcare team. A power of attorney for healthcare lets you appoint another person to make your healthcare decisions if you cannot speak for yourself. In other words, you are choosing someone to have the power to act in your place.

It is recommended that specialized, advance care planning is an essential component of patient-centered care for adults with chronic conditions or illness. Yet these conversations are often avoided by clinicians through fear of upsetting the patient, and they are often hindered by the uncertainty of their patient's prognosis.[20] While this process can be difficult, most individuals who have put an advance directive in place describe feeling a sense of relief once it is complete.

The process involves reflecting on what brings meaning and joy to your life, and deciding how you would want your medical treatment handled if you could no longer enjoy those things. Once you make these decisions you will need to share your wishes with loved ones and your care providers. The next step is to designate a healthcare agent or proxy (usually a close family member or friend) to carry out your wishes in the event that you are unable to communicate. For legal reassurance, this communication should be in writing in the form of an advance directive (advance directive forms can be accessed online), and the signed form can be copied and provided to both your healthcare institution as well as your healthcare proxy. This enables you to take control over what may happen in the future and to alleviate any related anxiety. It can also reduce conflict between family and healthcare providers at the end of life.

As difficult as it was to think about, once Bea completed her advance directive, she felt she had done the right thing. She wanted to be certain that her wishes were communicated clearly and that they would be followed should she ever become cognitively impaired and unable to speak for herself.

Goal Setting

Am I living in a way which is deeply satisfying to me, and which truly expresses me?
—Carl Rogers (1961)[21]

Goals give our lives a sense of purpose and meaning. It is important to have realistic goals to motivate us and keep us going across different areas of our lives such as relationship goals, career and educational goals, and those goals involving our hobbies and interests and personal growth. Throughout life our goals may shift and change for a multitude of reasons, but sometimes this is necessary following a change in our health status. While it is natural to feel sad if we have to let go of some goals, it's really important to replace or modify them so we still have plans, hope, and challenges in our lives. If your energy is limited, it can help to make sure you are using it wisely by focusing on what matters most to you.

Usually our goals are underpinned by our values and what is important to us. It can be helpful to take some time to think about your values and what matters to you across different areas of your life, such as the following[22]:

• Relationships (e.g., spending time with my family is important to me)
• Leisure and fun (e.g., learning how to paint is important to me)
• Work and education (e.g., being able to work part time matters to me)
• Personal growth (e.g., taking time to practice meditation matters to me)

You can then explore and set realistic goals for each area. It can help to break your goals down into more achievable steps.

Goal-Setting Exercise

S.M.A.R.T. criteria can help with goal setting; this involves the following steps[23]:

Specific—select a specific goal you want to work on (e.g., to learn to play the guitar).
Measurable—make sure progress is measurable (e.g., achieve Grade 1).
Assignable—state who will do it (e.g., you).
Realistic—make sure your goal is doable, given available resources (e.g., do you have access to a guitar and someone to teach you).
Time-related—state a deadline for achieving your goal (e.g., start lessons by the end of this month).

11

The Gifts of Congenital Heart Conditions

"You may not control all the events that happen to you, but you can decide not to be reduced by them."

—Maya Angelou, Letter to My Daughter[1]

In Kintsugi, the ancient Japanese mending practice, broken pottery is repaired by emphasizing the cracks with gold to represent healing, resilience, and restoration. This practice originates from the Buddhist philosophy Wabi Sabi, which centers on the acceptance and beauty of transience and imperfection. In the repaired pottery the wound is embraced, resulting in something more beautiful than the original.

Similarly, a solely negative focus on the impact of living with a congenital heart condition (CHC) provides a far from complete picture of this experience. Often survivors of traumatic experiences have been found to experience positive personal change, known as posttraumatic growth,[2] and enjoy an equal or better quality of life to their heart-healthy peers.

For many, being born with a heart condition puts the important things in life into perspective, often from infancy. Overcoming cardiac surgery or a medical crisis can make everyday worries seem insignificant. Witnessing who sticks by you through the various storms brings into focus who really matters, thus deepening meaningful relationships. Facing life threats can focus your sense of purpose, while a heightened awareness of the fragility of life can make you more grateful for each moment. Learning from infancy that life can be harsh builds resilience and perseverance. As such, many individuals report a greater appreciation for living life, the ability to develop closer relationships, increased empathy for others, and having a clearer view of what matters to them.

Many people who live with a disability report experiencing a high quality of life often in contrast to how they are perceived by observers, known as the "disability paradox." Studies have found that quality of life is dependent upon finding a balance among body, mind, and spirit while establishing and maintaining relationships, which many participants in their study, living with a disability, were able to achieve in contrast with social expectations.[3]

Posttraumatic Growth

Living with someone with CHC makes you more grateful for simple pleasures in life.
—Xavier, spouse, 52 years old, United States

The transformative power of suffering has been depicted in history, poetry, art, and literature throughout human history. More recently positive psychological transformation following stressful or traumatic events is referred to as posttraumatic growth. One study found that 90% of trauma survivors reported experiencing at least one aspect of posttraumatic growth after a stressful encounter.[4] Traits that seem to be helpful in the process of developing posttraumatic growth include good emotional regulation skills,[5] openness to trying new things, willingness to re-examine your belief system, meaning-making, and reaching out and connecting with others.[6]

Posttraumatic growth has been described as encompassing five broad areas: increased personal strength, changed priorities, more meaningful relationships, changed philosophies, and spiritual development.

Personal Strength

My scar is not who I am, but it is why I am. I am living proof of miracles, kindness, sacrifice, and hope. My scar tells a story and I am humbled to wear that story with pride.
—Rylee, 36 years old, United States

Posttraumatic growth can increase personal resilience, our "ability to bounce back" from stressful or traumatic experiences. Resilience is a process and can be an outcome of getting through trauma. Literature has shown that individuals with a CHC tend to be extremely resilient. Personal resilience enables us to work through problems, learn from challenging experiences, and feel motivated to achieve our goals. Self-awareness, an optimistic out-look, and having the coping skills to stay calm under pressure and regu-late our emotions can strengthen resilience. It is important to note that resilience isn't always about storming ahead and getting on with it. Just as importantly, it is about recognizing when you need to rest, recuperate, and heal. Resilience can be honed and developed; it is not something you do or don't have. Many of the techniques and tools we have described throughout this book aim to strengthen resilience. It is important to note that for each of us resilience has its limits and can diminish when stress becomes too overwhelming. After all, we are only human!

> *Recently I received treatment for breast cancer, and during this period many of the health-care professionals who attended to me commended me for my resilience, strength, and positive attitude. Personally I believe it's my CHD that has made me strong, has shown me that I can overcome more than I might think, and it has helped me find the freedom within myself to not get stuck in victimhood but look to the future with hope in my heart.*
> —Charlotte, 42 years old, The Netherlands

Generally, the CHC population has exceeded medical expectations in many ways: both in terms of physical health and, more broadly, with many individuals going on to not only survive but also thrive in life. This can occur when we compensate for what we cannot do by making the most of what we can do with a keen determination, perseverance, and motivation. Everyday problems that seem like mountains to our heart-healthy peers can seem like molehills to some of us.

In fact, many well-known public figures are thriving with a CHC, including US athlete Shaun White, born with tetralogy of Fallot, who has won several gold medals in Olympic snowboarding and skateboarding; Bian Littrel, singer from the Backstreet Boys, who was born with a ventricular septal defect; the British singer Jessie J, who has Wolff-Parkinson-White syndrome; and the British comedian Robert Webb, who was recently diag-nosed with a CHC at the age of 47.

Growing up "feeling different" can have its positives, too. When you are used to having to think things through from a unique perspective, it makes you less likely to just go along with everyone else and better able and more confident to problem-solve, "think outside the box," make your own deci-sions, and tolerate "standing out from the crowd."

Wisdom is also born out of difficult life experiences, and people with a CHC often demonstrate the wisdom of someone much older, often having experienced more obstacles in childhood than most do in a lifetime. Also, sometimes facing the absurdity of life can help you develop a keen sense of humor.

> *The success I have had is from true old-fashion grit, determination, and a fighting spirit. Never-give-up attitude. I see myself as a heart warrior and not as a survivor or victim. I have never let my "disability" be my excuse not to do things—yes, it has been challenging but always look for a way to succeed. I mountain bike—yes, I use an ebike but better than doing nothing. I swim, canoe, and enjoy life to the full. I have three sons and am self-employed and so living the best way I can—as a warrior. My suggestion to others is to fight, fight, fight the good fight of life, and live it to the full.*
>
> —Andrew, "Heart Warrior," 52 years old, South Africa

Changed Priorities

> *In gay culture, one is often led to believe that a perfect physique with six-pack abs is required to fit in. As a gay man with a CHD, complete with surgical scars on my body (and "hidden" abs), it can be easy to feel like I don't fit in or like I'm not "enough." I believe that my ability to overcome health expectations, as an avid cyclist and endurance event enthusiast, has truly helped me to embrace the fact that fitting in is no longer necessary, nor desired. I only aspire to live my best life for as long as I can.*
>
> —Ethan, 40 years old, United States

Many people with a CHC report that their life priorities are clearer and they can let go of life's little stressors more easily. Being reminded of what matters in life by surviving cardiac surgery, medical incidents, and other adversities can put smaller worries into perspective, liberate us from getting caught up in more superficial concerns, and enable us to enjoy life and appreciate the small things.

> *At 41 years old, Kyle had gone through two open heart surgeries, one as a child and again in his early 20s. He had a pacemaker implanted at the age of 28 which needs to be surgically replaced every 7 years or so. He became keenly aware at a very young age of how fragile life is and, as a result, works hard at creating a life that is meaningful. He takes excellent care of himself physically, spends a lot of time with family and friends, and worked hard to obtain a job he enjoys which allows him to give back to others. He prides himself on living in the moment and "not sweating the small stuff." Unlike his friends, growing older doesn't bother him one bit; in fact, he throws himself a birthday party each year and looks forward to touring twice a year on his motorcycle with his wife.*

More Meaningful Relationships

My sister's health challenges have been a constant reminder of the importance of family.

—Walter, 49 years old, United States

Survivors of adversity often respond with increased empathy, thus "becoming more human."[7] Experiencing suffering, pain, loss, and hardship and having to depend on others during periods of poor health can foster humility and enhanced awareness of the value of human connection. Further, witnessing the suffering of others, for example other children during hospital stays or appointments, makes us very aware of how difficult life can be for others, too. This insight can make us value others, feel more socially connected, and become less judgmental. Often this leads to a greater sense of altruism and prosocial behaviors. We may feel more driven to prevent others from suffering, explaining perhaps why so many of us are "wounded healers,"[8] who are drawn to the caring professions.

Enduring dramatic life events can also deepen meaningful relationships with our families, friends, and peers. In relationships, we are more able to let the small stuff go and focus on what really matters. Adversity is also associated with greater acceptance of self and increased self-expression. Living through a health crisis and dealing with chronic symptoms can also tell us who is able and willing to stand by us through the hard times. It tells us who is really prepared to be there for us when things get tough and often makes us feel deeply connected to those who do. This experience may teach us what it takes to be a close friend or trusted family member, and then, in turn, we may be more likely to give to others in a similar way.

Some of the most amazing people in my life I have met because we are connected through CHD—from moms of little kids with heart defects to people my age and older. It's wonderful to have people around who understand and have been where you are. People you can share your worries and fears with, people who will be there for you when you feel like your world is falling apart, people who will be the first ones cheering you on, and people who just get you and the emotional rollercoaster you are on for life. Thank you to the wonderful heart people in my life who just understand in a way nobody else ever will.

—PKH, 28 years old, Austria

Changed Philosophies

When I was first introduced to ACHA (Adult Congenital Heart Association) at the Peer Mentorship training, it was my first time to meet any other CHD adults. It was a wonderful experience and I found that we all have a lot in common on how we think about life. I have always been grateful for life. I believe most people take life for granted—the CHD community does not. We all seem to have a different way of thinking about life and living—we cherish our time.

—Denny, 67 years old, United States

Many people report experiencing new insights about their life and a renewed sense of purpose and direction following traumatic experiences. People with a CHC often note that they are determined to "make the most out of life" especially following cardiac surgery or a health crisis. They may refocus their plans and goals to align them with their values.

Further, we can be less likely to get "caught in the rat race" because we truly appreciate our health and well-being and how easily this can be lost; instead, we focus more on a healthy work–life balance to prioritize what really matters.

We know how to take each day as it comes, appreciating the good days and learning to be truly present in the moment.

Gemma didn't find out she had a congenital cardiac condition until she was 31 after collapsing at home. She required emergency open heart surgery. She was shocked to learn she had lived with the condition since birth. While she recovered from the surgery relatively quickly, it took some time to recover mentally and process what had happened to her. Over time, she completely reassessed her life, swapping her high-paid, demanding, and stressful job for something more rewarding, spending more time with her family and friends who had supported her during her recovery, and making sure she took care of herself. Although it wasn't without its challenges, in many ways she considered the CHC as a gift that had forced her to re-evaluate her life and focus on what really matters.

Spiritual Development

I've made it six decades due to quickly advancing medical capabilities, a great support system of family and close friends, and a strong faith. I firmly believe that I have survived and thrived for nearly 60 years with my CHD for a reason, and I take comfort in the hope that what has been learned from my case has in some way benefited others.

—Mitch, 59 years old, United States

Posttraumatic growth can also include developing a more positive perspective, a deeper appreciation of life, spiritual connection, and for some new or deeper religious beliefs. Individuals with a CHC often report feeling a profound sense of gratitude for their lives heightened by the knowledge of its fragility. Following periods of suffering they are better able to appreciate periods of greater health and less likely to take their well-being for granted.

> *Tricia spent her 30th birthday in the ICU (intensive care unit) after having an unexpected side effect from a cardiac procedure. While there she tapped into her religious side and prayed for a recovery and a life of "normal, everyday problems." She did recover and now 20 years later reminds herself of that time whenever she feels frustrated by bills, work stress, or arguments with her family. She also now loves and celebrates every birthday regardless of the number attached. That traumatic experience helped her sharpen her perspective on what is truly important and maintain a sense of ongoing gratitude.*

Following adversity people are often motivated to create meaning from their suffering and may express this creatively, for example through writing, painting, music, or other outlets, or feel compelled to contribute to positive change, for example through advocacy or charity work.

It is important to remember that it is not the case that some of us respond negatively to adversity while others remain strong and resilient. The same people who report posttraumatic mental health difficulties can also experience posttraumatic growth. These responses may become entwined, perhaps making it more difficult for others to understand and notice the hurt behind our stoicism.

Nurturing Posttraumatic Growth

Individuals can also deliberately develop posttraumatic growth.[9] Several factors are known to provide a pathway to healing and personal growth following adversity, including having the opportunity to share our story, to feel heard and understood by others and ourselves. This is one of the reasons that counseling or therapy can be helpful. Chatting with peers, reading similar biographical stories, and writing about our experiences can also be insightful and therapeutic for the same reason. Good social support and nourishing relationships can help to protect us from mental health problems, and having strong role models may inspire us and help us to focus on positive goals.

Another important factor is feeling empowered to manage some aspects of what is happening to us, particularly regarding our health (e.g., by having a good understanding of our condition and feeling heard by our medical care providers). The ability to manage and regulate our emotions is also associated with posttraumatic growth,[10] and we discuss developing emotional regulation skills in Chapter 6. Additionally, there is a growing body of evidence that has demonstrated the benefits of gratitude on our physical health and well-being, and it also helps to mitigate burnout.[11] "Gratitude interventions" such as keeping a "gratitude journal" can help us to develop posttraumatic growth.

Gratitude Journal

We realize that it can be challenging to remember all that you have to be grateful for, especially in the midst of a crisis. However, research has shown this can improve our overall mental health if practiced regularly.[12] Cultivating an overall sense of gratitude can help you to remain in the present and lower stress. It can also help to promote posttraumatic growth and well-being. There are several ways that you can incorporate this into your life. Look around you and notice all of the positive things in your life that bring you happiness. Be grateful for a sunny day, a comfortable place to rest, an ability to smell the flowers, or enjoy time with family or friends. Some people find it useful to keep a daily gratitude journal. Alternatively, others have focused on writing letters of gratitude to those who have been kind to them in the past. Some tips from the experts on getting the most out of keeping one include the following:

- Make a conscious decision to focus on positives in life.
- Become mindful of your day and the "small things," such as watching a beautiful bird fly by or enjoying the warm sunshine on your face.
- Build gratitude journaling into your days; even a new 5-minute habit can make a big difference.

Make a record in your journal of things that you genuinely feel grateful for in as much detail as possible (rather than just listing things for the sake of it). Try to practice this daily, if possible. It is okay if you repeat the items on your list.

At the sake of sounding cliché, I have found that acceptance of the things I cannot change and trying to live a full, authentic life has helped me tremendously in coping with my congenital heart disease. It's incredibly easy to dwell on the unknown, but I've found daily meditation and journaling have helped me maintain a more positive and hopeful outlook for the future that is centered on who I am apart from my congenital heart disease. I have renewed old passions and found new ones that have allowed me to shape an identity that includes my congenital heart disease but is not defined by it.

—*Nicole, 36 years old, United States*

Choose Happy

Research suggests that we can incorporate everyday activities into our day-to-day life to promote happiness.[13] We have listed some of the main activities researchers have found to make people happier in Table 11.1.

My heart and all of its complications have always made me feel special. There are times when I prefer to live in ignorance of how serious my condition is, and there are times when I take a step back and accept my life and limitations and feel proud of how far I've come and how much I'm trying to keep going.

—*Mia, 40 years old, United States*

As CHD survivors, many of us were not meant to live beyond a certain age in childhood. Today, we are teachers, doctors, mothers, actors, Olympians, artists, people in our communities and of the world—living our best lives. My scar is a reminder of how precious life is and a symbol of the love, care, and commitment of individuals and communities that I have met and have been surrounded with all of my life: from the healthcare providers who saved and supported my life, to my family, friends, teachers, and advocates who look out for me and share with me all of life's experiences. I do get caught up with the worries and pressures of life. So to slow down every now and then, I reach for the (fuchsia) stethoscope that I got for myself shortly after my fourth open heart surgery 9 years ago. Listening to my own special heartbeat brings a comfort and a sense of awe and gratitude. My CHD shows me that I can live life gently, with reverence and thankfulness. It is this lesson and the sense of community that I am grateful for.

—*Nina, 39 years old, born and raised in Malaysia*

Table 11.1 Find Happiness . . .

- Start with the basics: get enough sleep, eat nourishing food, hydrate, and get some sunshine
- Engage in activities where you are able to lose yourself, termed "flow"
- Find an activity you enjoy that doesn't involve money, technology, alcohol, or drugs
- Pay attention to and savor life's joy—revisit the good times in your mind or look through happy photographs
- Spend time in nature
- Practice acts of kindness and smile
- Visualize positive outcomes
- Nurture your meaningful relationships; call, text, or write to an old friend
- Learn to forgive and let resentments go; avoid rumination
- Practice good self-care. Schedule a date with yourself each week
- Avoid "compare and despair," overthinking, or social comparison
- Establish and commit to your goals (see previous exercise)
- Develop new strategies for coping
- Make plans you can look forward to
- Start a gratitude journal
- Give to others through volunteerism
- Be a lifelong learner
- Surround yourself with happy people, positive podcasts, and comedies
- Adopt a pet or a plant to care for

12

Supporting People with a Congenital Heart Condition

A Guide for Loved Ones

While living with a congenital heart condition (CHC) can, at times, be challenging, it can be just as hard when you love someone with a CHC. Whether you are a parent, spouse, sibling, or friend, we applaud your commitment to your loved one and recognize, at times, it can seem like a rollercoaster, with many ups and downs. One of the most helpful things you can do for your loved one is to take care of yourself. You simply can't pour from an empty cup, and if you don't take care of your own needs, you may end up burnt out. Your self-care is essential, and you may also benefit from many of the tools and techniques described throughout Chapters 5–8. We have also outlined other ways you can support your loved ones here.

> *Growing up with a sister with CHC, I didn't know, realize, or understand the seriousness of it all. It was just part of our life. The doctor's appointments, hospital stays, surgeries, etc. She didn't look or act sick, so I honestly never thought of her as sick. As an adult and mother, it hits me like a ton of bricks what my sister has endured her whole life, and I am heartbroken for what she has dealt with and continues to deal with. I think family therapy would have been very helpful for all of us. However, when I look at her now, I still don't see sickness: I see courage, strength, pride, and complete admiration.*
>
> —*Marie, 51 years old, sister, United States*

Supporting Loved Ones

- Always look past their condition to see them.

- Gain an understanding of their condition by having knowledge of their CHC and how it can affect them. This will help you to be in a more informed position to support them.
- Do not take on a "martyr's role" as no one should have to take on all of the stress and responsibility associated with caring for a loved one during times of poor health.
- Don't nag, criticize, or lecture.
- Do not stay silent when you have something important to say.
- Be mindful to not "smother" them and help them retain their independence and contribution to family life, as possible.
- Support them to Pace, Plan, and Prioritize their time and energy (see Chapter 9).
- Listen and validate (don't minimize) the difficulties they face.
- Often we want to fix things for people we care about, but often this is not possible, and it is enough to just be there and sit with them.
- Work with them and help them focus on achievable goals.
- Keep communicating; open and honest conversations are key to avoiding misunderstandings and resentments.
- Take steps to recognize and manage your own emotional distress (draw from Chapters 5–8).
- Recognize if you need breaks or support; reach out to your wider support network. No single person can meet all of our needs.
- Allow them to find ways to give back; reciprocity is essential for healthy relationships.

Getting through Medical Crisis

Over the many years that we have been together, my wife has been through lots of medical crises which have impacted on our family life. I have always tried to stay calm for her while focusing on keeping things as normal as possible for our son.

—Jamie, 45 years old, spouse, United Kingdom

When someone you care about is experiencing an acute period of illness, hospitalization, surgery, or a long period of recovery, it can cause emotional, physical, and financial strain. You may need to drive your loved one to multiple appointments, cover double childcare and household duties, or spend countless hours at your loved one's bedside. It is easy to become overwhelmed during medical emergencies, with the hospital experience itself and the uncertainty that comes with surgery and the road to recovery. If that is the case, we urge you to remember to take care of yourself by being aware of your simple, basic physical needs.

- Make sure that you stay well hydrated.
- Eat meals (even if you don't have an appetite).
- Try to get adequate sleep.
- Make sure you get a break from the hospital.
- Take some time to take a shower, get changed, and refresh.
- Try to ensure some physical movement (e.g., a walk on the hospital grounds or to the gift shop).
- If weather permits, get outside every day.

These tasks seem simple, but when you are dealing with a hospitalization or with someone who is seriously ill, it can be hard to remember. However, it is vital to keep your strength up and avoid burnout and compassion fatigue.

Assemble a Team

During my friend's lengthy hospital stay, I tried to visit her as regularly as possible to provide my support. I found her high level of patience and resilience incredible. When she had to go into hospital, we were all very worried about her, but it was important to be calm for her child and provide support to keep his routine as normal as possible as this was clearly her top priority.

—Friend, United Kingdom

Essentially, we urge you not to try to do it all yourself. When you have the chance to gather your thoughts, it can help to make a list of you and your loved one's needs so that when friends, neighbors, or family ask how they can help, you will have this list on hand with tasks. If you need help with childcare, assistance with meal preparation, or want someone to come and stay with your loved one so you can take a break, identify who is able to fill that role and assign them to it. Perhaps it is too difficult keeping up with calls and texts from concerned family members; you could assign someone to start a line of communication. With that in place, you can rest assured that those who need the information will get it while you can focus your efforts on caring for your loved one and yourself. Following we have listed some ways others may be helpful to you and your loved one:

- Coordinate meal preparation
- Childcare and carpooling

- Pet care
- Research on locating specialists, if needed
- Rides to and from the hospital or doctor's appointments
- Calling family and friends
- Getting mail
- Visiting with your loved one
- Watering plants; house and garden maintenance

We've learned that most people want to be given a task to help. Otherwise, they may feel helpless or left out of what is going on. Asking for help doesn't come easy to everyone, but it is essential when you are going through a medical crisis. You may even find that asking for assistance can deepen your relationships, and that your loved ones will feel more comfortable coming to you when they are in need in the future.

Following are some things to avoid:

- Minimizing the situation by saying "It could be worse."
- Avoiding talking about the medical situation for fear of making them (the family member who is currently unwell) feel worse.
- Sharing their health information with others without their consent.
- Leaning on them emotionally for your own reassurance.
- Avoiding them because you don't know what to say.
- Excluding them from your plans for fear of asking them to overdo it.

Following are some things you could say:

- I am here for you.
- How can I help?
- Do you need me to listen, or do you want me to help you problem-solve what to do next?

What You Can Do for Your Loved One in the Hospital

- Help them get comfy and ensure their basic needs are met (bringing comforting items, clothing, toiletries, drinks, treats, books, magazines, etc.).
- Pay attention to what the healthcare professionals are saying and take notes. Ask for clarification of anything you or your loved one doesn't understand.
- Offer to accompany them to doctor's appointments.

- Be available if they need a shoulder to cry on.
- Manage visitors and provide updates (or get a second-in-command to field them).
- Help them to focus on positive memories, plans for the future, and good news.
- Recognize that medical staff are human and are not all-knowing.
- Stay calm when dealing with your loved one's healthcare providers.
- Become the information coordinator if your loved one is unable to.
- Remember that coping with a CHC affects everyone in the family. Observe how all of the members of your family are coping and check in with them occasionally.
- Help secure additional support for those members of the family who may need it (remember self-care, too).
- Assist with financial management, and let educators or employers know about the current situation.

Where to Get Help

- The point person in the Adult Congenital Heart Disease (ACHD) center (physician's assistant or an advanced nurse practitioner)
- Patient advice and liaison officer (United Kingdom)
- Accommodation liaison officer (United Kingdom)
- Hospital social worker (United States) or psychologist
- Hospital chaplain

Dealing with Medical Staff

As the mother of a CHC baby, who is now in her 40s, I learnt to not be intimidated by medical professionals or for that matter anyone, from cleaners to professors. I suffered a lot of pain before I learned not to let it bother me or what they thought of me. When my baby was born very poorly, I was desperate for information, asking many questions of anyone who came to check her; unfortunately some gave me the wrong information instead of admitting they didn't know. All that matters is your precious child, who no one knows like you do, even as an adult.

—Elizabeth, parent of an adult with CHC, 72 years old, United Kingdom

Often caregivers and loved ones feel a conflict between worrying about burdening medical staff and wanting to advocate for the needs of their loved one when they are hospitalized or unwell. Healthcare professionals can be very busy, and it can be difficult to get the time to ask them questions or find out essential information. Our key message is that you should not worry about being a nuisance. While, of course, it is important to always be polite and courteous, your priority is your loved one and you know them best. Communicating calmly and assertively is important (you may benefit from reading the section on "Assertive Communication" in Chapter 8), and if you have any questions or concerns about their care, you have a right to raise them and to be afforded time to discuss them.

A Guide for Healthcare Professionals

First, we want to thank you for dedicating years of your life to learning how to care for us and then committing to doing so. For holding our hand as we count back from 10 and drift unconscious pre-surgery, tending our wounds, and dabbing our brow as we recover. For helping us steady ourselves back on our feet, finding humor with us in the, at times, absurdity of life with a CHC and interpreting our electrocardiograms, X-rays, and pacemaker interrogations. Thank you for sharing good news with us and wiping our tears when the outcome is more difficult. We want to thank those who advocate and fight for us and who literally touch our hearts. You share our joy when we are discharged and when we reach milestones. Never underestimate the importance of the work you do and how much you matter to us. Living with a lifelong heart condition can be challenging, and our healthcare team is very much part of our "heart family."

Psychologically Informed Medicine

My husband and I were just teenagers when our daughter (now in her 50s) was born. When she was going through her surgeries, her medical team became our family. Her doctor was more than just a doctor; she was a surrogate mother to all of us. That place was home.

—Mae, mother, 73 years old, United States

As described extensively throughout this book (which we strongly encourage you to read), those of us living with a lifelong heart condition can face a multitude of unique life stressors, as a direct and indirect result of our condition. Lifetime prevalence of depression, anxiety, and posttraumatic stress disorder (PTSD) for adults with a CHC is as high as 50%,[1] and currently the mental health needs of this population are poorly met. While many of the life challenges that contribute to these mental health outcomes are unavoidable (such as the need for cardiac surgery, medical tests, and emergency procedures), it is important for you to know that there are many ways to mitigate their impact and to promote protective factors and positive adaptation.

Grounding medical care in the most recent psychologically informed, holistic understanding will help to enable us to live as normal a life as possible. Here we describe what has been termed " Psychologically Informed Medicine,"[2] an approach that aims to minimize mental health risk factors and to promote protective factors within the healthcare setting. This approach comprises promoting compassionate-reflective practice, a soothing presence, social inclusion, and trauma-informed practice.

Compassionate–Reflective Practice

First, it is important to recognize the power imbalance between the healthcare professional and the patient.[3] Within this relationship dynamic there exists an imbalance of power in health status, medical knowledge, and access to often lifesaving medical care. Often there are also socioeconomic disparities in terms of education, social status, and finances. This imbalance can be exacerbated by disempowering aspects of care such as being asked to wear a backless hospital gown or being clinically held during medical procedures.[4] At our most vulnerable, as a patient, we have little choice but to entrust our life to our medical team. In this "patient role," we may feel vulnerable, dependent, frightened, and disempowered. This can result in a loss of agency, which can prevent us from articulating our concerns, asking key questions, or remembering what has been said after clinical encounters. It is important to recognize and reflectively navigate this imbalance of power to facilitate trust, mutual respect, and dignity, and to avoid paternalism, especially for a population who depend on medical care from "cradle to grave." This is important because feeling disempowered and not listened to by healthcare providers can increase risk of psychological distress and the development of medically related PTSD, and it can impact negatively on adherence to medical recommendations and attendance at appointments.

> *Even though I consider myself to be very health literate, able to understand my own complex heart condition and navigate the health system, I often find myself feeling somewhat numb following annual checkup appointments with my cardiologist. Before I know it, the consult is over, my questions remain unanswered, and I'm already outside the hospital or clinic with more uncertainty than before the appointment, with at least another year before I will have the opportunity to ask the questions again, suspended in uncertainty and concern about my health.*
>
> —*Benjamin, 39 years old, Australia*

Successfully negotiating this power imbalance to engender trust can be achieved through empathic and compassionate communication, within the context of a boundaried professional relationship. Feeling psychologically safe is central to mental health, well-being, and the development of trust.[5] For social beings, psychological safety is often relational and communicated through compassion.[6] One study found that feeling safer during the process of hospitalization increased feelings of control, calm, and hope.[7]

In other words, the human factor is essential to quality health and social care provision. Historically often left to the "bedside manner" of the individual healthcare professional, it is increasingly recognized that communication skills are a core aspect of patient care that can and should be taught across all training programs and as continual professional development, throughout the career journey, for all medical healthcare professionals.[8]

> *It takes a lot for many of our patients to trust us, given their understandable anxiety and sometimes poor previous experiences with healthcare. It's a real challenge to maintain communication through that, to demonstrate a commitment to working through that as a patient/healthcare team, and nothing is more rewarding than a patient learning to trust you.*
>
> —*ACHD cardiologist, United Kingdom*

Compassionate communication is not just about improving the patient's psychological and emotional experience. These "soft skills" have demonstrable outcomes, with studies reporting improved survival rates when doctors make eye contact and provide reassuring touch to their patients.[9] Simply put, what you say when we are at our most vulnerable matters more than you may ever realize.

To feel as psychologically safe as possible, we need to be able to trust that healthcare providers understand the limits of their competencies and will reach out to specialist colleagues as required. We understand that we are often medically complex, with our care needs dependent on the cutting edge of medical knowledge. Many of us have lived with medical uncertainty from day one. We are more likely to fear someone who lacks the required expertise who is not listening to us or "having a go" (there is every chance we have already had bad experiences of this and are fearful of it happening again) than admitting that they need to reach out to another specialist colleague for support. Please listen to us, too. We have a lifetime of experience and might be able to help or direct you to who does have the information that may make a difference in our medical outcome. It is important that our lived experience is acknowledged and validated, with any concerns being taken seriously.

By proactively working to make us feel more comfortable and at ease, we will feel safer and more empowered to express our concerns, process and recall important information, and thereby feel in control of our lifelong healthcare journey. Providing accessible information, avoiding the use of medical jargon, checking to ensure that we have understood, taking seriously any concerns, and making time to answer any questions are essential components of facilitating healthcare literacy and self-management of chronic health conditions.

Of course, fundamental to a compassionate-reflective approach is recognition of the challenging work healthcare professionals do and the emotional and psychological impact this can have. Providing clinical supervision could help to alleviate this burden and help to prevent moral injury and burnout.[10] We strongly advocate for psychologists and clinical social workers (United States) to be embedded within the medical team not only to support patients but also to offer supervision and support to healthcare staff, as a way of reducing the stress and burden of your high-demand jobs.

You may also benefit from exploring and drawing on the tools and techniques covered in Chapters 5–8 of this book.

During my Fontan surgery, two anesthesiologists and the entire cardiac team were in the OR (operating room) with me for over 14 hours. Doctors sat next to my ICU (intensive care unit) bed and prayed during the 3 days I was in a drug-induced coma and my parents couldn't see me. Nurses braided my hair and cared for me. I know God and my grandmother were watching over me.

—*Rylee, 36 years old, United States*

Recommendations

- Hospitals and our medical team are likely a significant and consistent part of our lives and hold unique meaning and purpose for us. We probably have mixed feelings about this because despite being associated with feeling unwell and perhaps pain and trauma, they also offer us hope, treatment, safety, and sanctuary. Our healthcare journey is lifelong; as such, every medical encounter matters.
- Always see the person; whether we are conscious or not, in a hospital gown or bed, asking for a commode or pain medication. We are not just patients; we are fellow human beings, perhaps someone's parent, son, daughter, friend, or colleague. In a different time or place, you or yours could find themselves in our position.
- Please listen to us; we know our own bodies. We may have had similar experiences before, and we may be able to help. Please work in partnership with us.
- Please be careful not to imply blame when something goes wrong, such as pacing or implantable cardioverter-defibrillator (ICD) leads coming loose.
- If you are not a specialist, please consult with our usual specialist care providers as soon as possible (or someone with specialist adult congenital heart disease [ACHD] knowledge of our condition). We need to trust you are working within your competencies.
- Please understand if we are a bit irritable or not our best selves; we may be in pain, frightened, and feeling powerless. When you meet us, we are probably at our most vulnerable.
- Words matter. Please always be sensitive to our situation and try not to say things like "You must be used to this." You don't get used to pain, discomfort, and fear; if anything, difficult past experiences can make it even more challenging.
- Please avoid showing your excitement when you hear our rare diagnosis. Please don't say things like "Wow, you look so much better in person than you do on paper."
- If you are unsure of what the best treatment plan is, tell us that. Schedule a timely follow-up with us so that you can take your time and consult with others in the field.

- Be careful not to deny our bodily experience by saying things like "But other people with this condition don't feel like this." We need you to listen and validate what we are experiencing.
- Avoid and challenge derogatory, stigmatizing labels such as "twiddler" (of pacing device), "sick role," "difficult/challenging patient," "frequent flyer," "lost cause," or "attention seeker."
- Give your patients an easy way to communicate with the team in case they have follow-up questions.
- Advocate for integrative mental health services as part of your ACHD team.
- Find a way to make testing a bit easier for us. For instance, enable us to listen to music during our cardiopulmonary stress test, watch a comedy during our echocardiogram, and not have extensive wait times before our appointments.
- Find a way to balance between being honest with your patients while also offering some degree of hope. Many of us were saved by the cutting edge of technology in the 11th hour, and technology continues to change rapidly.
- Refer to and encourage cardiac exercise rehabilitation when appropriate, bearing in mind the dramatic changes in exercise recommendations and that some adults with a CHC may be anxious about pushing themselves because it conflicts with previous advice to restrict activity.
- Don't avoid or dismiss the difficult conversations, such as advance care planning, genetic counseling, sexual health, transplant, and getting older. Your patient may want to discuss these issues and be worrying alone about them. It is important they are sensitively addressed as part of care.
- Understand if your patient would like to seek a second opinion. Some of us have the experience of having our cardiac care mismanaged, and sometimes we just need some additional reassurance before proceeding with a new treatment. We get this is your career, but please remember this is our life.
- Introduce, recommend, and bring humor into your life and your practice.
- Take care of yourself. Self-care is an essential part of being a caregiver or healer. It will help to prevent burnout, moral injury, compassion fatigue, and vicarious trauma. It will also help you to be clear-minded when making important decisions about patient care.

Soothing Presence and Social Inclusion

Research suggests that the soothing presence of a loved one can mitigate ad-verse medical experiences. It is well established that social support is one of the most protective factors for our mental health and well-being. The reassuring touch and voice of a loved one can facilitate a feeling of safety and comfort across the lifespan. Research studies have demonstrated that touch facilitates the tasks of the vagus system by expressing compassion and providing feelings of reward, reciprocity, and safety.[11] To illustrate, skin-to-skin contact, such as kangaroo care, has been shown to reduce mortality, severe illness, infection, length of hospital stay, improves sleep organization and modulation of pain responses in preterm babies,[12] while preterm infants gain significantly more weight when they are touched.[13] Compassion is also expressed through vocal-ization;[14] for example, a recent study found that maternal speech decreases pain and increases oxytocin levels in preterm infants during painful procedures.[15]

Therefore, we strongly advocate for the presence of loved ones to be fa-cilitated as much as possible throughout the patient journey. For example, enabling a partner to stay overnight on a cot or recliner following their surgery and having open-access visits during hospital stays, as possible. Each hospital has their own regulations around overnight stays and visiting hours, and many have had to restrict them, unfortunately, during acute phases of the COVID-19 pandemic.

> *We look after many of our patients lifelong, and it's an incredible privilege to get to know patients and their families over many years.*
> *—ACHD cardiologist, United Kingdom*

Consistency of care from familiar medical staff is also important.[16] We need to be able to build a trusting relationship with our care team, and this is not possible if we see a different healthcare provider at every appoint-ment. Having a named point of contact, such as a specialist nurse, can help. Generally, consistency of care remains a challenge for adults for whom care provision can be inconsistent and difficult to access, calling for improved service provision, consistency of care, and the development of healthcare standards to this end.[17]

> *I was one of the first to go through the transition from pediatrics to the new adult service. It was very daunting going from my childhood hospital where I spent many years and*

knew well. I knew everyone in each department from phlebotomy to echo then back to the ward. I was seen by my new cardiologist at pediatrics first, and she then continued to see me at the adult clinic so it was nice to have familiarity. I had known all those involved in my care very well, and it's the thing I find most difficult about my (adult) care now. I try to get to know my clinicians and feel connected, which is hard when you don't see the same person.

—*Ailsa, 36 years old, United Kingdom*

The growing number of people living with a congenital heart condition (CHC) has created a relatively new population, which, coupled with the often hidden nature of this condition, can lead to limited understanding and awareness in wider society. Despite being the most common congenital condition, CHCs remain relatively poorly represented, understood, and supported in wider society, with many individuals lost to care. This is arguably a public health crisis that merits public health campaigning involving people with lived experience to ensure adequate representation of the unique challenges faced by this population.

As healthcare professionals, you have a unique opportunity to promote awareness and advocate for improved support among allied health professional colleagues (such as general practitioners, dentists, midwifery teams) and beyond; please do. Working in partnership with wider systems, such as schools, patient groups, and workplaces, to improve awareness and understanding should improve social inclusion and quality of life.

Recommendations

- Consider rules around the presence of loved ones in the medical setting, for example enabling a partner to stay overnight with open-access visits during hospital stays, as possible.
- Promote and advocate for improved awareness and social inclusion.
- Be sure to advocate for patient-centered care, which includes collaborating with nonspecialists and partnering with your patients and their family members.

Trauma-Informed Practice

I went to the emergency room (ER) with another episode of atrial arrhythmias and went home with an implantable cardiac defibrillator (ICD) implanted in my chest

muscle. Nobody mentioned how painful it would be or how it would affect my life. Of
course I'm grateful, but this is when I could have used some counseling, which wasn't
available.

—Sandra, Canada, 59 years old

Individuals with a CHC are often exposed to invasive medical interventions, which can be painful and frightening. They may cause feelings
of helplessness, give a sense of life threat,[18] and contribute to feelings of
anxiety and trigger symptoms of posttraumatic stress.[19] Cardiac medical
events can be uniquely abrupt and unexpected, leading to emergency
trips to the hospital, as in the cases of certain arrhythmias, heart failure,
device failure, stroke, and cardiac arrest. Living with a CHC can involve living with uncomfortable physical symptoms and/or uncertain
diagnoses and involve routine exposure to a range of diagnostics tests
and invasive procedures such as pacemaker or ICD implant, ablation, or
cardiac surgery.[20] It is perhaps not surprising then to find an increased
risk of developing post traumatic stress disorder (PTSD) in the CHC
population, considering we are often exposed to the perfect storm of
risk factors which may result in what has been termed cardiac-induced
PTSD (CI-PTSD).[21]

Feeling powerless is a risk factor for PTSD, and as part of a psychologically informed approach, it is essential that the healthcare system better addresses disempowering aspects of care across the patient journey to support
health, well-being, recovery, and our trust in those who care for us.

Following my third surgery, the heartbeat I had been used to for my entire life was no
longer audible and had been replaced by the click of a mechanical valve. After having
three sternotomies (in childhood, as a teenager, and as an adult) the shape of my chest
has been impacted. Having abrupt changes to physiology has been more difficult than
what could have been anticipated. Making patients aware of these changes (particularly
younger patients) is something that would have been beneficial to me. This could be part
of broader, integrated psychosocial support.

—Benjamin, 39 years old, Australia

It can help to take time to explore our wishes prior to invasive or painful
medical procedures. Informing and engaging us in making choices about
these procedures, including ensuring adequate pain management, asking
what matters to us, and facilitating coping techniques such as distraction or
the presence of a loved one can also help to mitigate the psychological impact. It can be difficult to distinguish between benign cardiac arrhythmias

and more serious issues, especially if similar feelings in the past have indi-cated a serious problem, which can lead to heart-focused health anxiety.[22] Understanding this and taking the time to validate and explore our con-cerns will help us manage our condition.

During hospital stays, we are often exposed to unnecessary disruptions to sleep and recovery when we need it most. The hospital setting can be stressful, exposing us to loud noises such as heart monitors, harsh lighting, poor privacy, and multiple awakenings. Often this is established to suit the shift pattern of the attendant medical or cleaning staff rather than through medical necessity. Researchers suggest that this atmosphere may contribute to a transient increase in vulnerability to further episodes of hospitalization termed "post-hospital syndrome."[23] The development of a more healing environment by addressing these factors could improve patient experience and, psychological and medical outcomes.

> *When hospitalized, the beeping on the heart monitor in Rebeccah's room is a trigger to her PTSD. She always asks the medical staff to turn the volume lower or off completely. Sometimes they will and sometimes they won't. When they lower the volume, it makes a huge difference in how she is feeling emotionally.*

It is also important to address depersonalizing aspects of care such as hospital gowns, especially given that patients are frequently being asked to wear them even when there is no medical reason for them to do so.[24] CHC patients report associating the backless hospital gown with symbolic embodiment of being in the patient role, relinquishing control to medical professionals, and feelings of physical and emotional vulnerability. Further, many struggle to put it on themselves and report that it limits activity and changes how they see themselves. It is important its use is limited to med-ical necessity and other, less revealing, designs are considered.

Providing patients with a copy of clinical letters, access to their clinical notes, and involving them in aspects of their care may also help to ad-dress any power imbalance between patients and medical professionals and enable self-management and a sense of autonomy and control over their condition. It is essential that we are provided with a summary, handheld (if online portals are not available, or if the patient is unable to access it) copy of our medical notes and care plan in case of emergency or, for example, if we are traveling out of our local area.

Waiting for different aspects of healthcare can add to the burden of living with a lifelong condition.[25] For example, during outpatient visits we may have to wait for appointments, tests, test results, and phone calls, and as inpatients, we may, for example, wait for surgery and to be discharged. Hospital satisfaction and social attitude surveys repeatedly find that access and waiting times are a major source of dissatisfaction for patients, reason for complaints, and an indicator of poor-quality care. We know that aspects of patient care that contribute to feelings of powerlessness, such as excessive waiting, can increase psychological distress. It is essential that waiting time across the patient journey is addressed.

Please be sensitive about asking us to be available as a "training case" for trainee healthcare professionals during medical appointments and hospital stays. It is likely we have been asked this many times before, since infancy. We have heard of and personally experienced this being taken for granted without permission being sought. This is not okay; we must be asked to consent to this in advance sensitively so as not to reinforce our sense of being a "medical curiosity," especially when we are at our most vulnerable. Of course, we want to contribute to medical teaching, but we also need to always be seen as a person with agency and a right to privacy. The same applies to the use of our medical history or information as an interesting "case discussion," for example at a conference, in an academic article, or on social media.

As mentioned previously, a CHC specialist psychologist or clinical social worker (in the United States) should be embedded within the healthcare team to promote psychological well-being across the life course.[26] Access to appropriate and timely psychological support is simply essential for this cohort. Furthermore, fostering links between medical and psychological care and patient support groups could encourage peer-to-peer support and improve wider social support.[27]

Recommendations

- Try to keep the hospital environment peaceful and "healing" focused; minimize loud noises such as laughter, chat, noisy shoes, doors or bins slamming shut, or constant beeping heart monitors. Reconsider harsh lighting as possible.
- Consider whether disruptions to a sleeping patient are essential, such as waking patients up to take very early morning observations because this time fits around a change in staff shifts.

- It can be hard living with a lifelong heart condition. Coming back to the hospital can trigger previous traumatic experiences (e.g., being held down for clinical procedures). Even if we are fully grown adults, we may need a loved one beside us.
- If they are required at all keep the use of backless hospital gowns to medical necessity. If possible, find a more dignified alternative.
- Be mindful of waiting across the patient journey, which includes appointments, phone calls for surgery slots, tests, results, and discharge. Please minimize this as much as possible.
- As an inpatient, small things are a very big deal when you feel unwell, vulnerable, and helpless, such as waiting on someone to help you change from a hospital gown into your pajamas, for pain relief, for a commode, or to refill your water jug when you are bed bound. Try not to keep patients waiting for basic needs.
- Systemic inefficiencies such as repeatedly being asked by multiple healthcare professionals for your medical history are exhausting when you feel unwell; please read our notes first.
- Please ensure clear communication with others involved in our care so tests and procedures are not repeated unnecessarily.
- Please be sensitive about our history; ask for consent before presenting us to trainees as an "interesting case" or sharing our information with others, even anonymously (many of us are so medically unique it would be quite easy to infer identity).
- Provide adequate sensitivity training to the frontline administrative staff who answer the telephone, schedule the appointments, and greet patients as they arrive for their outpatient appointments, assist with weight checks, and so on. Keep in mind how impactful each of these "touch points" can be in relaying care, connection, and calm.

Questions to Ask Your CHC Patient to Support Mental Health and Well-Being

- How are you feeling generally?
- Do you have any concerns about your health and well-being?
- Does thinking about your health make you feel worried, low, or afraid?
- What is important to you?
- Would you like to discuss longer-term health outcomes?

- Do you have someone to talk to about your concerns?
- Would you find it useful to have someone to talk to?
- It is understandable if you feel overwhelmed because you have a lot to deal with. How can we help?

A Guide for Mental Health Professionals

In my early 30s I found a body psychotherapist who transformed my life. I was at breaking point, and she was the first healthcare professional to acknowledge that the experiences I endure as a result of my CHC are far from normal. By validating my feelings she made me recognize that I am not "crazy"; rather, I was experiencing a normal response to a lifetime of abnormal experiences. I stopped fighting against my body and pushing myself to function like everyone else. I began to accept my condition, look after myself, and become more empowered regarding my health needs.
—Beth, 44 years, United Kingdom

Astoundingly, lifetime prevalence of depression, anxiety, and PTSD for adults with a CHC is currently as high as 50%.[28] People living with a CHC are often interested in psychological treatment, but there is currently underrecognition and undertreatment of mental health concerns.[29] Mental health professionals have a role to play in advocating for the mental health needs of this population both by working therapeutically with individuals with a CHC and by promoting psychologically informed practice across the wider healthcare community. When working with this community, it is important to validate and understand the very real psychosocial challenges we face and to carefully navigate therapeutic intervention without further pathologizing a normal response to multiple lifelong adversities. As such, we encourage you to read this book in full to gain a more comprehensive understanding of these challenges while holding in mind that every individual with a CHC will have a unique experience and story to tell.

It is vital to recognize the oppressive impact of discrimination and ableism experienced by people living with a heart condition from birth and how this impacts negatively on mental health. Often people experiencing this are unaware of the hidden barriers themselves or may have internalized discrimination, impacting negatively on self-esteem and identity. Considering this oppression with an awareness of intersectionality with other inequalities such as race and gender is essential to understanding the diverse lived experience of people with a CHC. Further, cultural and religious beliefs can impact on the experience of living with a congenital condition, such as attitudinal or financial barriers to accessing healthcare and social stigma, so it is important to take this into account too.

It is important to be aware of the more common issues that clients with a CHC history may present with, such as the following:

- Identity, feeling different, low self-esteem, body image, and scarring
- Cardiac-induced PTSD, medical, and body trauma
- Feeling disempowered (e.g., as a result of being in the patient role, bullying or social exclusion, or difficulty accessing specialist care)
- Loss (e.g., of a normal childhood, being able to have children)
- Adjustment to a decline in health
- Preparing for further medical monitoring and interventions (cardiac device implant, open heart surgery, ablation, transplant)
- Living with medical events (e.g., arrhythmias, potential ICD shock) and medical uncertainty
- Managing chronic physical symptoms, such as pain and fatigue
- Any negative impact on relationships, education, careers, finances, and life choices
- Impact of having a CHC on primary caregivers, siblings, children, and family dynamics
- Feeling overwhelmed about the impact of cumulative medical interventions, events, and life stressors
- Historically poor access to psychological support for the client or their family

I have had a traumatic few years with atrial flutter and felt very frustrated, angry, and scared. Never in my life has my heart condition ruled what I have done as much as it did then. I have had no mental health support despite seeking help.
—Ailsa, 36 years old, United Kingdom

Given the high prevalence of PTSD and the potential exposure to medical trauma in the CHC population, such individuals may benefit from trauma-informed psychological interventions that incorporate safety and stabilization strategies with a holistic understanding.[30] A relational stance with a focus on compassion to challenge any hypervigilance to threat or body trauma and to develop self-soothing strategies may also be beneficial.[31] It is also important to recognize resilience factors and positive adaptation, which may mask more difficult psychological responses yet, when utilized carefully, can be drawn on to facilitate healing, coping, and empowerment.

> *We had no counseling or psychological help. As a family, it was a very lonely experience, I would recommend that you seek professional help; there is no shame in needing it.*
> —Elizabeth, *parent of an adult with a CHC, 72 years old, United Kingdom*

Some of the medications commonly used for cardiac patients, including beta blockers and digoxin, could contribute to psychiatric symptoms. This is something that you or your individual client may want to speak with their ACHD specialist about if it is suspected as a possibility.

Recommendations for Mental Health Professionals

- Recognize that while there are common themes, every client has a very different story to tell; even clients with the same condition will likely have experienced a different journey.
- Validate and understand the extensive psychosocial challenges this population can face without further pathologizing a normal response to multiple lifelong adversities.
- Recognize if this normative response has developed into a more serious mental health condition such as anxiety, depression, PTSD, complex PTSD, or an eating disorder (especially if there are issues with body image).
- Be aware of the medical historical context of your client. It is important to understand that the healthcare they may have received growing up may be vastly different to what is currently available. Consider what this may mean in terms of exposure to medical trauma; attachment; pain relief; a lack of access to play therapy or psychological support; predicted prognosis; and the impact on education, physical activity, and social inclusion (see Chapters 1–4).
- Develop a therapeutic alliance through empathetic understanding; avoid pity.
- Evaluate coping skills and help the client build new healthy strategies, if needed.
- Assess for substance misuse (including prescription drugs such as opioids and/or benzodiazepines).
- Be aware of the increased use of denial as a defense mechanism.

- Focus on empowering your client to build skills to assert their needs and to self-advocate in order to better manage their condition.
- For clients with a trauma history, incorporate safety and stabilization strategies with a holistic understanding.
- Encourage and contain emotional release and processing to help the client develop emotional regulation skills.
- Assess the need for grief work and address it, as appropriate.
- Address any issues around identity, low self-esteem, and body image (screen for eating disorders, self-harm, suicidality, or risk-taking behaviors).
- Help your client to develop and focus on realistic, value-driven goals.
- Assist your client in anxiety reduction in preparation for upcoming procedures or surgeries.
- Empower your client to take an active role in managing their healthcare.
- Use evidence-based treatments, as appropriate to your level of training and competencies. While evidence is emerging, some that have been found to be helpful in adults with CHC include (trauma-informed) cognitive behavioral therapy (CBT), eye movement desensitization and reprocessing (EMDR) therapy, acceptance and commitment therapy (ACT), body psychotherapy, and mindfulness-based stress reduction treatments.
- Encourage peer support through hospital-based groups, patient support organizations, or online platforms.
- Be open to working with family members and significant others, as needed.
- Seek regular consultation, as needed. Address your own issues around serious illness, pain, and mortality.
- Recognize strengths building on resilience and posttraumatic growth while being mindful that positive adaptation may mask psychological distress.
- Recognize the impact and interaction between discrimination and ableism on life choices, social inclusion, representation and mental health.
- Consider intersectionality and the impact of social, cultural, and religious beliefs, for each individual.
- Advocate for better awareness, understanding, and support of the psychological needs of the CHC population and integrative psychology

services as part of ACHD teams. Educate other health and social care professionals involved in their care about the unique psychological needs of the CHC population.

- If you are involved in research, bear in mind this is a population who have been objectified and studied from birth. As such, try to meaningfully include people with lived experience when considering the priorities and design of your study and ensure any findings are accessible and disseminated back to the CHC population.

Afterword

We are humbled by all of the encouragement we received for writing this book from so many of you in the congenital heart community, and we are grateful to the exceptional individuals who shared their personal experiences for the purposes of this book. We are filled with hope that the contents of this book will be helpful to many of you. Perhaps you already knew about the history of congenital heart conditions (CHC), but really needed to learn some new stress reduction exercises. Maybe you are a family member wanting to increase your understanding of your loved one's experience or a healthcare professional looking to better meet the needs of your patients. Or perhaps you are an individual with a CHC, and after reading this book you are able to feel a bit less alone in your lived experience. Whatever your situation may be, we hope that reading this book is a step in a positive direction toward feeling more connected and that it will help you to live your best life.

We realize that despite all that we have learned in the process of writing this book, we still have a lot to learn. By the time that this book comes off the press, there will most likely be new and exciting developments in the fields of congenital cardiology and mental health. We expect and hope that there will be innovative research and a continuous flow of cutting-edge technology to offer new solutions to our healthcare challenges. We are excited about the prospects of this growing field and future breakthroughs. We are also hopeful this book will contribute to better recognition of the wider psychological and social impact of living with this serious, lifelong medical condition, and a more holistic approach in meeting the needs of our CHC community. Thank you for engaging with our work, and we wish you hope, strength, and love in your CHC journey. (For photos of our personal experiences with CHC, see Figures A.1–A.5.)

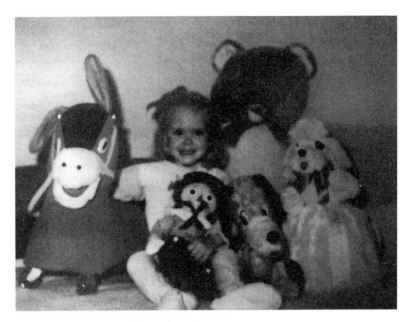

Figure A.1 Tracy's hospital homecoming.

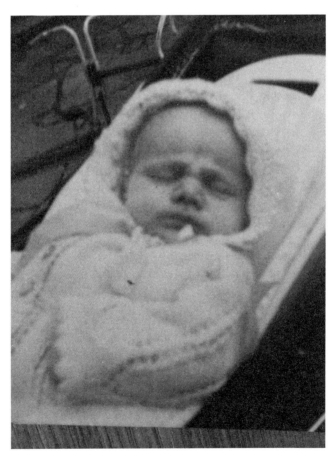

Figure A.2 Liza's first day home from hospital at 6 weeks old, Scotland.

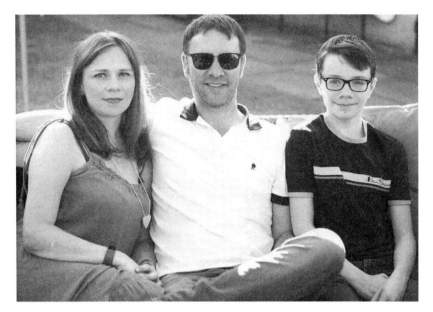

Figure A.3 Liza with her husband, Craig; and their son, Dylan.

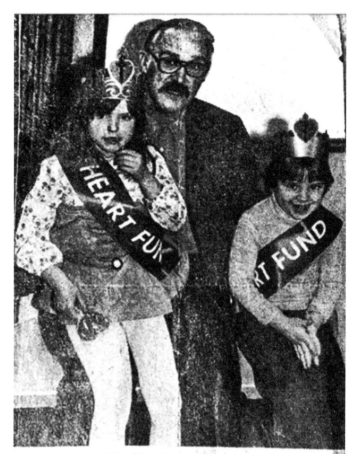

TAKING HEART—Six-year-old Tracey Kustwan and Steve Franklin, 5, chosen as the official prince and princess of the Westfield Heart Fund Drive, are living proof of some of the medical miracles accomplished through Heart Association research. Both children, pictured above with pediatrician Dr. George Flessas have undergone heart operations made possible only in recent years through Heart Association research backed by Heart Fund dollars. The annual fund drive will be kicked off Wednesday. On Heart Sunday, Feb. 24, volunteers will go door-to-door asking for contributions.　　(Evening News

Figure A.4 Tracy as heart princess, *Westfield Evening News*.

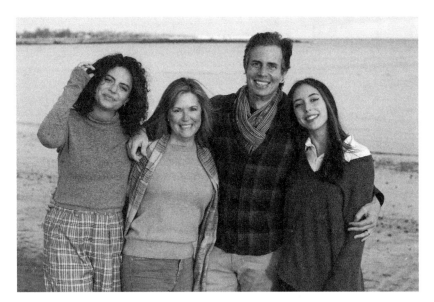

Figure A.5 Tracy with her husband, Joe; and their daughters, Sophia and Grace.

Appendix: Useful Organizations and Resources

Congenital Heart Condition Patient–Advocacy Support Organizations

Australia

- The Heart Foundation (https://www.heartfoundation.org.au/)

Canada

- Canadian Adult Congenital Heart Network (http://www.cachnet.org/)
- CCHA for Life (https://www.cchaforlife.org/)

United Kingdom

- Arrhythmia Alliance (http://www.arrhythmiaalliance.org.uk/)
- The British Heart Foundation (https://www.bhf.org.uk/)
- Chest Heart and Stroke Scotland (https://www.chss.org.uk/)
- Little Heart Matters (single ventricle) (https://www.lhm.org.uk/)
- Somerville Heart Foundation (https://sfhearts.org.uk/)

United States

- Adult Congenital Heart Association (https://www.achaheart.org)
- Children's Heart Foundation (https://www.childrensheartfoundation.org/)
- Congenital Heart Public Health Consortium (CHPHC) (https://www.aap.org/en/patient-care/congenital-heart-defects/congenital-heart-public-health-consortium/)

- Conquering CHD: https://www.conqueringchd.org/about/about-cchd/
- Mended Hearts (https://mendedhearts.org/connect/)

Global Outreach

- Children's Heart Link (https://childrensheartlink.org/)
- Global ARCH (https://global-arch.org/)
- International Society for Adult Congenital Heart Disease (https://www.isachd.org/home)

Other Useful Resources

Congenital Heart Condition Organizations

- Asia Pacific Society for ACHD (http://www.apsachd.org)
- Association for European Paediatric and Congenital Cardiology (https://www.aepc.org/)
- British Association for Congenital Cardiac Nurses Association (https://baccna.org.uk/)
- British Cardiovascular Society (https://www.bcs.com/)
- British Congenital Cardiac Association (https://www.bcca-uk.org)
- Congenital Cardiac Anesthesia Society (https://ccasociety.org/)
- Congenital Cardiac Nursing Association (UK) (http://www.ccn-a.co.uk/)
- Congenital Cardiology Today (https://www.congenitalcardiologytoday.com/)
- Congenital Heart International Professionals' Network (CHIP) (https://thechipnetwork.org/)
- Congenital Heart Surgeons Society (https://chss.org/)
- ECHDO—European Congenital Heart Disease Organisation (https://www.echdo.eu/)
- Global Alliance for Rheumatic and Congenital Hearts (Global ARCH) (https://global-arch.org/)
- Heart Kids SA (South Africa) (https://www.heartkids.co.za/index.html)
- Iranian Society of Pediatric Cardiology (http://www.ispc.ir/en)
- Japanese Society for ACHD (http://www.jsachd.org/)
- Johns Hopkins All Children's Heart Institute (https://www.hopkinsallchildrens.org/services/heart-institute)

- North American ACHD program
- Pediatric and Congenital Electrophysiology Society (https://www.pace sep.org/)
- Pediatric Cardiac Society of India (http://www.pediatriccardiacsociety ofindia.com/)
- Pediatric Cardiac Society of South Africa (http://www.pcssa.org/)
- Pan Arab Congenital Heart Disease Association (https://aubmc.org.lb/)
- World Society for Pediatric and Congenital Heart Surgery (WSPCHS) (https://wspchs.org/)

Healthcare Guidelines

- AHA Scientific Statement: Psychological Outcomes and Interventions for Individuals with Congenital Heart Disease: A Scientific Statement from the American Heart Association https://www.ahajournals.org/doi/epdf/10.1161/HCQ.0000000000000110
- AHA/ACC ACHD Guidelines (2018) (https://www.ahajournals.org/doi/10.1161/CIR.0000000000000603)
- American College of Cardiology and the American Heart Association at https://www.ahajournals.org/doi/pdf/10.1161/CIR.0000000000000603. For a shorter summary of the main points, please visit: https://www.acc.org/~/media/Non-Clinical/Files-PDFs-Excel-MS-Word-etc/Guidelines/2018/Guidelines_Made_Simple_Tool_2018_ACHD.pdf
- England, Wales, and Northern Ireland (https://www.england.nhs.uk/wp-content/uploads/2018/08/Congenital-heart-disease-standards-and-specifications.pdf)
- ESC ACHD Guidelines (2020) (https://www.escardio.org/Guidelines/Clinical-Practice-Guidelines/Grown-Up-Congenital-Heart-Disease-Management-of)
- ESC GUCH Working Group Advance Care Planning Guidelines (2020) (https://www.escardio.org/Guidelines/Clinical-Practice-Guidelines/Grown-Up-Congenital-Heart-Disease-Management-of)
- Scotland (National) Congenital Heart Disease Specialist Standards— SCCS (https://www.sccs.scot.nhs.uk/2018/01/31/congenital-heart-disease-specialist-standards/)
- Scotland (National Standards for Local Care)—Congenital heart disease standards (https://www.healthcareimprovementscotland.org/our_work/standards_and_guidelines/stnds/chd_standards.aspx)

Adult Congenital heart Association Accreditation Criteria

- https://www.achaheart.org/media/3471/accreditationprogramcriteria2022.pdf

Travel Resource

- List of US-accredited centers (https://www.achahe art.org/your- heart/resources/clinic-directory/)
- The ACHA Travel Directory (international)—https://www.achaheart.org/media/3080/traveldirectory13thedition.pdf

Mental Health Organizations

International

- This directory lists contact information for national associations of psychology around the world: https://www.apa.org/international/networks/organizations/national-orgs#c

United States

- American Foundation for Suicide Prevention: https://afsp.org
- The American Psychological Association: https://www.apa.org/
- The National Alliance on Mental Illness: https://nami.org/Home
- The National Association for Social Workers: https://www.socialworkers.org
- Psychology Today: https://www.psychologytoday.com/us

United Kingdom

- The British Association of Behavioural and Cognitive Psychotherapies (BABCP): https://babcp.com/
- The British Association for Counselling and Psychotherapy (BACP): https://www.bacp.co.uk/
- The British Psychological Society: https://www.bps.org.uk/public/find-psychologist
- The Health and Care Professions Council (HCPC): https://www.hcpc-uk.org/check-the-register/

Notes

PREFACE: OUR HOPE AND MISSION

1. Sutton, J. 2015. "Scars as a celebration of life: Jon Sutton reports on a new exhibition led by Dr Liza Morton, who then gives her perspective." *The Psychologist 8*: 185; Morton, L. 2015. "Scars as a celebration of life." *The Psychologist 28*: 185.
2. 1942, Dust Tracks on a Road: An Autobiography by Zora Neale Hurston.
3. Dasmahapatra, H. K., M. P. Jamieson, and G. M. Brewster. 1986. "Permanent cardiac pacemaker in infants and children." *Thoracic Cardiovascular Surgery 34*: 230–235; Reid, J. M., E. N. Coleman, and W. Doig. 1982. "Complete congenital heart block: Report of 35 cases." *British Heart Journal 48*: 236–239. Morton L. The heart of medicine: growing up with pioneering treatment BMJ 2015; 351: h3881 doi:10.1136/bmj.h3881
4. Weinreb, S. J., O., Okunowo, H. Griffis, and V. Vetter. 2022. "Incidence of morbidity and mortality in a cohort of congenital complete heart block patients followed over 40 years." *Heart Rhythm* February 22: 1149–1155. doi:10.1016/j.hrthm.2022.02.019. PMID: 35217197.
5. Morton, L. 2019. "NHS needs to learn how people living with serious heart disease feel about it." *The Scotsman,* October; Freeman, T. 2014. "The heart of the issue: Interview with Liza Morton." *Holyrood, Scotland's fortnightly political and current affairs magazine,* February 19.
6. Matter, M., H. Almarsafawy, M. Hafez, G. Attia, and M. Magdy Abou Elkier. 2011. "Balloon atrial septostomy: The oldest cardiac interventional procedure in Mansoura." *Egyptian Heart Journal 63* (2): 125–129.
7. Frank Arthur W. 1995. The Wounded Storyteller: Body Illness and Ethics. Chicago: University of Chicago Press.
8. Stapleton, C. M., H. Zhang, and J. S. Berman. 2021. "The event-specific benefits of writing about a difficult life experience." *Europe's Journal of Psychology 17* (1): 53–69.

CHAPTER 1

1. Ooues, G., P. Clift, and S. Bowater. 2018. "Patient experience within the Adult Congenital Heart Disease Outreach Network: A questionnaire-based study." *Journal of Congenital Heart Disease 2* (7). https://doi.org/10.1186/s40949-018-0020-3.

2. Ntiloudi, D., M. A. Gatzoulis, A. Alexandra, H. Karvounis, and G. Giannakoulas. 2021. "Adult congenital heart disease: Looking back, moving forward." *International Journal of Cardiology Congenital Heart Disease 2*. https://doi.org/10.1016/j.ijcchd.2020.100076.

3. Gatzoulis, M. A., L. Swan, J. Therrien, and G. A. Pantley. 2010. *Adult congenital heart disease: A practical guide*. 2nd ed. Blackwell.

4. Perloff, J. K. 1973. "Pediatric congenital becomes a postoperative adult: The changing population of congenital heart disease." *Circulation 47*: 606–619.

5. Greatbatch, W. 2000. *The making of the pacemaker*. Prometheus Books.

6. "What happened when a baby girl got a heart transplant from a baboon." 2015. *Time*, October 26.

7. Gatzoulis, Swan, Therrien, and Pantley 2010.

8. Spector, L. G., J. S. Menk, J. H. Knight, C. McCracken, A. S. Thomas, J. M. Vinocur, M. E. Oster, J. D. St Louis, J. H. Moller, and L. Kochilas. 2018. "Trends in long-term mortality after congenital heart surgery." *Journal of the American College of Cardiology 71* (21): 2434–2446. doi:10.1016/j.jacc.2018.03.491.

9. GBD 2017 Congenital Heart Disease Collaborators. 2020. "Global, regional, and national burden of congenital heart disease, 1990–2017: A systematic analysis for the Global Burden of Disease Study 2017." *The Lancet Child and Adolescent Health 4* (3): 185–200. https://doi.org/10.1016/S2352-4642(19)30402-X.

10. Chen, M., T. Riehle-Colarusso, and L. F. Yeung. 2018. "Children with heart conditions and their special health care needs—United States." *Morbidity and Mortality Weekly Report 67*: 1045–1049.

11. Liu, Y., S. Chen, L. Zühlke, G. C. Black, M. Choy, N. Li, and B. D. Keavney. 2019. "Global birth prevalence of congenital heart defects 1970–2017: Updated systematic review and meta-analysis of 260 studies." *International Journal of Epidemiology 48* (2): 455–463. https://doi.org/10.1093/ije/dyz009.

12. Gatzoulis, Swan, Therrien, and Pantley 2010.

13. Morton, S. U., D. Quiat, J. G. Seidman, and C. E. Seidman. 2021. "Genomic frontiers in congenital heart disease." *Nature Reviews Cardiology*. https://doi.org/10.1038/s41569-021-00587-4.

14. Congenital Heart Public Health Consortium. 2019. "Know the facts." Congenital Heart Defect Fact Sheets. https://www.aap.org.

15. Vilchinsky, N., K. Ginzburg, K. Fait, and E. B. Foa. 2017. "Cardiac-disease-induced PTSD (CDI-PTSD): A systematic review." *Clinical Psychology Review 55*: 92–106. https://doi.org/10.1016/j.cpr.2017.04.009.

16. Verrall, C., G. Blue, A. Loughran-Fowlds, N. A. Kasparian, K. Walker, S. Dunwoodie, G. F. Sholler, and D. S. Winlaw. 2019. "'Big issues' in neurodevelopment in congenital heart disease." *Open Heart*. doi:10.1136/openhrt-2018-000998.

17. St Pierre, A., P. Khattra, M. Johnson, L. Cender, S. Manzano, and L. Holsti. 2010. "Content validation of the Infant Malnutrition and Feeding Checklist for Congenital Heart Disease." *Journal of Pediatric Nursing 25*: 367–374.

18. Wilson, W. M., M. Smith-Parrish, B. S. Marino, and A. H. Kovacs. 2015. "Neurodevelopmental and psychosocial outcomes across the congenital heart

disease lifespan." *Progress in Pediatric Cardiology 39*: 113–118.; Wernosky, G., K. M. Stiles, K. Gauvreau, T. L. Gentles, A. J. du Plessis, and D. C. Bellinger. 2000. "Cognitive development after the Fontan operation." *Circulation 102*: 883–889.

19. Horner, T., R. Liberthson, and M. S. Jellinek. 2000. "Psychosocial profile of adults with complex congenital heart disease." *Mayo Clinic Procedures 75*: 31–36.

20. Livecchi, T. 2004. "Psychosocial issues affecting adults with congenital heart disease: One patient's perspective." *Nursing Clinics of North America 39* (4): 787–789. doi:10.1016/j.cnur.2004.08.003.

21. Morton, L. 2020a. "Using psychologically informed care to improve mental health and wellbeing for people living with a heart condition from birth: A statement paper." *Journal of Health Psychology 25* (2). https://doi.org/10.1177/1359105319826354.

22. Aquilina, A. 2006. "A brief history of cardiac pacing." *Images in Paediatric Cardiology 8* (2): 17–81.

23. Dasmahapatra, H. K., M. P. Jamieson, and G. M. Brewster. 1986. "Permanent cardiac pacemaker in infants and children." *Journal of Thoracic and Cardiovascular Surgery 34*: 230–235.

24. Morton 2020a.

25. iSupport Team. 2021. "Getting it right first time and every time; re-thinking children's rights when they have a clinical procedure." *Journal of Pediatric Nursing 61*: A10–A12. https://doi.org/10.1016/j.pedn.2021.11.017.

26. Anand, K. J., and P. R. Hickey. 1987. "Pain and its effects in the human neonate and fetus." *New England Journal of Medicine 317*: 1321–1329.

27. Morton 2020a.

28. Ezzeddine, F. M., T. Moe, G. Ephrem, and W. A. Kay. 2019. "Do we have the ACHD physician resources we need to care for the burgeoning ACHD population?" *Congenital Heart Disease 14* (4): 511–516. https://pubmed.ncbi.nlm.nih.gov/30945809/.

29. Morton, L. 2019. "NHS needs to learn how people living with serious heart disease feel about it." *The Scotsman*, October.

30. GBD 2017 Congenital Heart Disease Collaborators. 2020. "Global, regional, and national burden of congenital heart disease, 1990–2017: A systematic analysis for the Global Burden of Disease Study 2017." *The Lancet Child and Adolescent Health 4* (3): 185–200. https://doi.org/10.1016/S2352-4642(19)30402-X.

31. Stout, K. K., C. J. Daniels, J. A. Aboulhosn, B. Bozkurt, C. S. Broberg, J. M. Colman, S. R. Crumb, et al. 2019. "2018 AHA/ACC guideline for the management of adults with congenital heart disease: Executive summary: A report of the American College of Cardiology/American Heart Association Task Force on Clinical Practice Guidelines." *Circulation 139* (14): e637–e697. doi:10.1161/CIR.0000000000000602; Greutmann, M., D. Tobler, A. H. Kovacs, et al. 2015. "Increasing mortality burden among adults with complex congenital heart disease." *Congenital Heart Disease 10*: 117–127.

32. Congenital Heart Public Health Consortium 2019.

33. Wray, J., A. Frigola, and C. Bull. 2012. "Loss to specialist follow-up in congenital heart disease; out of sight, out of mind." *Heart 99* (7): 485–490.

34. Landzberg, M. J., and M. Gurvitz. 2018. "Transition education: Formative steps, in need of direction." *Journal of the American College of Cardiology 71* (16): 1778. doi:10.1016/j.jacc.2018.03.004.

35. Said, S. M., D. D. Driscoll, and J. A. Dearani. 2015. "Transition of care in congenital heart disease from pediatrics to adulthood." *Seminars in Pediatric Surgery 24*: 69–72.

36. Mackie, A. S., R. Ionescu-Ittu, J. Therrien, L. Pilote, M. Abrahamowicz, and A. J. Marelli. 2009. "Children and adults with congenital heart disease lost to follow-up: Who and when?" *Circulation 120* (4): 302–309. doi:10.1161/CIRCULATIONAHA.108.839464.

37. Hunter, A. L., and L. Swan. 2016. "Quality of life in adults living with congenital heart disease: Beyond morbidity and mortality." *Journal of Thoracic Disease 8* (12): E1632–E1636. doi:10.21037/jtd.2016.12.16.

38. Moons, P., S. Skogby, E.-L. Bratt, L. Zuhlke, A. Marelli, and E. Goossens. 2021. "Discontinuity of cardiac follow-up in young people with congenital heart disease transitioning to adulthood: A systematic review and meta-analysis." *Journal of the American Heart Association 10* (6, March).

39. Stout, K. K., C. J. Daniels, J. A. Aboulhosn, B. Bozkurt, C. S. Broberg, J. M. Colman, S. R. Crumb, et al. 2019. "2018 AHA/ACC guideline for the management of adults with congenital heart disease: Executive summary: A report of the American College of Cardiology/American Heart Association Task Force on Clinical Practice Guidelines." *Circulation 139* (14): e637–e697. doi:10.1161/CIR.0000000000000602.

40. EAPC, Sports Cardiology & Exercise Section of the European Association of Preventive Cardiology, ESC, European Society of Cardiology, and AEPC, Association for European Paediatric and Congenital Cardiology. 2020. "Recommendations for participation in competitive sport in adolescent and adult athletes with Congenital Heart Disease (CHD): Position statement." *European Heart Journal.* https://academic.oup.com/eurheartj/article/41/43/4191/5897398

41. Webb, G., M. J. Landzberg, and C. J. Daniels. 2014. "Specialized adult congenital heart care saves lives." *Circulation 129* (18): 1795–1796. doi:10.1161/CIRCULATIONAHA.114.009049.

CHAPTER 2

1. Van-Bulck, L., K. Luyckx, E. Goossens, and Moons P. 2021. "Identity formation in adults with congenital heart disease: What have we learned so far?" *International Journal of Cardiology Congenital Heart Disease.* https://doi.org/10.1016/j.ijcchd.2021.100183.

2. Moons, P., and K. Luyckx. 2019. "Quality-of-life research in adult patients with congenital heart disease: Current status and the way forward." *Acta Paediatrica. 108* (10): 1765–1772. doi:10.1111/apa.14876. PMID: 31136004.

3. Moons, P., and T. M. Norekvål. 2006. "Is sense of coherence a pathway for improving the quality of life of patients who grow up with chronic diseases? A hypothesis." *European Journal of Cardiovascular Nursing 5* (1): 16–20.

4. Calhoun, L. G., and R. G. Tedeschi. 2004. "The foundations of posttraumatic growth: New considerations." *Psychological Inquiry 15* (1): 93–102.

5. GBD 2017 Congenital Heart Disease Collaborators. 2017. "Global, regional, and national burden of congenital heart disease, 1990–2017: A systematic analysis for the Global Burden of Disease Study." *The Lancet Child and Adolescent Health 4* (3): 185–200.

6. Ladak, L. A., D. Pearson, K. Jenkins, M. Amanullah, W. Ahmad, K. D. Schmeck, A. Verstappen, and B. S. Hasan. 2020. "Adult congenital cardiac life-long needs evaluation in a low-middle income country, Pakistan." *Journal of the Pakistan Medical Association 70* (12): 2332–2338. doi:10.47391/JPMA.013.

7. Lopez Barreda, R., A. Guerrero, J. C. de la Cuadra, M. Scotoni, W. Salas, and F. Baraona. 2020. "Poverty, quality of life and psychological wellbeing in adults with congenital heart disease in Chile." *PLoS ONE 15* (10). https://doi.org/10.1371/journal.pone.0240383.

8. Liu, Y., S. Chen, L. Zühlke, G. C. Black, M. Choy, N. Li, and B. D. Keavney. 2019. "Global birth prevalence of congenital heart defects 1970–2017: Updated systematic review and meta-analysis of 260 studies." *International Journal of Epidemiology 48* (2): 455–463. https://doi.org/10.1093/ije/dyz009.

9. Adugna, M. B., Nabbouh, F., Shehata, S., et al. 2020. "Barriers and facilitators to healthcare access for children with disabilities in low and middle income sub-Saharan African countries: A scoping review." *BMC Health Services Research 20:* 15.

10. Morton, L. 2020b. "Ableism in psychology, every choice has been dictated by my health condition." *The Psychologist 33* (6).

11. Liu, Chen, Zühlke, Black, Choy, Li, and Keavney 2019.

12. McGrath, L., M. Taunton, S. Levy, A. Kovacs, C. Broberg, and A. Khan. 2020. "Abstract 16947: Barriers to care in urban and rural dwelling patients with adult congenital heart disease." *Circulation 142* (3): 142.

13. Jenkins, K. J., and M. A. Honein. 2018. "Public health approach to decrease mortality for congenital heart defects: Dying too soon." *Journal of the American College of Cardiology 71* (21): 2447–2449. doi:10.1016/j.jacc.2018.03.489.

14. Lopez Barreda, Guerrero, de la Cuadra, Scotoni, Salas, and Baraona 2020.

15. Bliss for Babies Born Premature or Sick. 2022. "Locked out: The impact of COVID-19 on neonatal care." Division of Clinical Psychology, British Association of Perinatal Medicine, Paediatric Critical Care Society and Association of Clinical Psychologists UK, 2022. "Open letter regarding continued restrictions on family visiting within paediatric and neonatal intensive care."

16. Bowlby, J. 1969. *Attachment and loss.* Basic Books.

17. Rothschild, B. 2000. *The body remembers: The psychophysiology of trauma and trauma treatment.* WW Norton & Company.

18. Livecchi, T. 2004. "Psychosocial issues affecting adults with congenital heart disease: One patient's perspective." *Nursing Clinics of North America 39* (4): 787–789. doi:10.1016/j.cnur.2004.08.003.

19. Dempster, N., C. L. Cua, G. Wernovsky, et al. 2017. "Children with hypoplastic left heart syndrome have lower quality of life than healthy controls and children with other illnesses." *Cardiology in the Young 28* (1): 1–6; Kovacs, A. H., A. S. Saidi, E. A. Kuhl, et al. 2009. "Depression and anxiety in adult congenital heart disease: Predicots and prevalence." *International Journal of Cardiology 137:* 158–164; Verstappen, A., D. Pearson, and A. H. Kovacs. 2006. "Adult congenital heart disease: The patient's perspective." *Cardiology Clinics 24:* 515–529.

20. Steiner, J. M., A. Dhami, C. E. Brown, K. K. Stout, J. R. Curtis, R. A. Engelberg, and J. N. Kirkpatrick. 2021. "It's part of who I am: The impact of congenital heart disease on adult identity and life experience." *International Journal of Cardiology Congenital Heart Disease 4.* https://doi.org/10.1016/j.ijc chd.2021.100146.

21. Verrall, C., G. Blue, A. Loughran-Fowlds, N. A. Kasparian, K. Walker, S. Dunwoodie, G. F. Sholler, and D. S. Winlaw. 2019. "'Big issues' in neurodevelopment in congenital heart disease." *Open Heart.* doi:10.1136/openhrt-2018-000998.

22. Gong, C. L., H. Zhao, Y. Wei, et al. 2020. "Lifetime burden of adult congenital heart disease in the USA using a microsimulation model." *Pediatric Cardiology.* https://doi.org/10.1007/s00246-020-02409-9.

23. Sluman, M. A., A. Apers, J. K. Sluiter, K. Nieuwenhuijsen, P. Moons, K. Luyckx, A. H. Kovacs, et al. 2019. "Education is important predictor for successful employment in adults with congenital heart disease worldwide." *Congenital Heart Disease 14* (3): 362–371.

24. Morton, L. 2020b. "Ableism in psychology: Every choice has been dictated by my health condition." *The Psychologist 33* (6).

25. Mackie, A. S., R. Ionescu-Ittu, J. Therrien, L. Pilote, M. Abrahamowicz, and A. J. Marelli. 2009. "Children and adults with congenital heart disease lost to follow-up: Who and when?" *Circulation 120* (4): 302–309. doi:10.1161/ CIRCULATIONAHA.108.839464.

26. Delaney, A. E., J. M. Qiu, C. S. Lee, K. S. Lyons, J. A. Vessey, and M. R. Fu. 2021. "Parents' perceptions of emerging adults with congenital heart disease: An integrative review of qualitative studies." *Journal of Pediatric Health Care 35* (4): 362–376; Lipstein, E. A. 2006. "Helping 'vulnerable' children—and their parents—lead normal lives: Vulnerable child syndrome distorts parents' perceptions of their child's health, disrupts the parent-child relationship, and can harm development and behavior in an otherwise healthy child." *Contemporary Pediatrics 23* (6).

27. Van-Bulck, Luyckx, Goossens, and Moons 2021.

28. Morton, L., N. Cogan, S. Kornfält, Z. Porter, and E. Georgiadis. 2020d. "Baring all: The impact of the hospital gown on patient wellbeing." *British Journal of*

Health Psychology 25 (3). doi.org/10.1111/bjhp.12416; Cogan, N., L. Morton, and E. Georgiadis. 2019. "Exploring the effect of the hospital gown on well-being: A mixed methods study." *The Lancet: Public Health, Special Issue* S32. https://doi.org/10.1016/S0140-6736(19)32829-6.

29. Meentken, M. G., I. M. van Beyman, J. S. Legerstee, et al. 2017. "Medically related post-traumatic stress in children and adolescents with congenital heart defects." *Frontiers in Paediatrics* 5 (20).

30. Deng, L. X., A. M. Khan, D. Drajpuch, et al. 2016. "Prevalence and correlates of post-traumatic stress disorder in adults with congenital heart disease." *American Journal of Cardiology* 1 (117): 853–857.

31. Weinreb, S. J., O. Okunowo, H. Griffis, and V. Vetter. 2022. "Incidence of morbidity and mortality in a cohort of congenital complete heart block patients followed over 40 years." *Heart Rhythm*, February 22: 1149–1155. doi:10.1016/j.hrthm.2022.02.019. PMID: 35217197.

32. Vieira, C. M., O. H. Franco, C. G. Restrepo, and T. Abel. 2020. "COVID-19: The forgotten priorities of the pandemic." *Maturitas 136*: 38–41.

33. Cogan, N., C. Kennedy, Z. Beck, L. McInnes, G. MacIntrye, L. Morton, J. Kolacz, and G. Tanner. 2021. "*ENACT project: Understanding the risk and protective factors for the mental wellbeing of health and social care workers in Scotland: Adapting to the challenges and lessons learned.*" Poster session presented at NHS Research Scotland Annual Scientific Meeting 2021: Adaption and renewal: Navigating our recovery, United Kingdom.

34. Cousino, M. K., S. K. Pasquali, J. C. Romano, M. D. Norris, S. Yu, G. Reichle, R. Lowery, S. Viers, and K. R. Schumacher. 2021. "Impact of the COVID-19 pandemic on CHD care and emotional wellbeing." *Cardiology in the Young 31* (5): 822–828. https://doi.org/10.1017/S1047951120004758; Morton, L., Calderwood, C., Cogan, N., Murphy, C., Nix, E., and Kolacz, J. 2022. "An exploration of psychological trauma and positive adaptation in adults with congenital heart disease during the COVID-19 pandemic." *Patient Experience Journal 9* (1): 82–94. doi:10.35680/2372-0247.1638.

35. Morton, L., N. Cogan, C. Calderwood, E. Nix, and J. Kolacz. 2021b. "Learning from adults with a lifelong congenital heart condition: Promoting post traumatic growth and mental health during COVID-19." Conference abstract from Trinity Health and Education International Research Conference 2021 (THEconf2021): "Transforming healthcare in a changing world: New ways of thinking and working."

36. Kovacs, A. H., A. S. Saidi, E. A. Kuhl, et al. 2009. "Depression and anxiety in adult congenital heart disease: Predicots and prevalence." *International Journal of Cardiology* 137: 158–164.

37. Stewart, J. C., and B. L. Rollman. 2014. "Optimizing approaches to addressing depression in cardiac patients: A comment on O'Neil et al." *Annals of Behavioral Medicine: A Publication of the Society of Behavioral Medicine 28* (2): 142–144. https://doi.org/10.1007/s12160-014-9615-x.

38. Horner, T., R. Liberthson, and M. S. Jellinek. 2000. "Psychosocial profile of adults with complex congenital heart disease." *Mayo Clinic Proceedings 75*: 31–36.
39. Horner, Liberthson, and Jellinek 2000.
40. Kovacs, A. H., A. S. Saidi, E. A. Kuhl, et al. 2009.
41. Westhoff-Bleck, M., J. Briest, D. Fraccarollo, D. Hilfiker-Kleiner, L. Winter, U. Maske, M. Busch, S. Bleich, J. Bauersachs, and K. Kahl. 2016. "Mental disorders in adults with congenital heart disease: Unmet needs and impact on quality of life." *Journal of Affective Disorders 204*: 180–186.
42. Khawaja, I. S., J. J. Westermeyer, P. Gajwani, and R. E. Feinstein. 2009. "Depression and coronary artery disease: The association, mechanisms, and therapeutic implications." *Psychiatry (Edgmont) 6* (1): 38–51.
43. Edmondson, D., I. M. Kronish, J. A. Falzon, and M. M. Burg. 2013. "Posttraumatic stress disorder and risk for coronary heart disease: A meta-analytic review." *American Heart Journal 166* (5): 806–814. https://doi.org/10.1016/j.ahj.2013.07.031.
44. DiMatteo, M. R., H. S. Lepper, and T. W. Croghan. 2000. "Depression is a risk factor for noncompliance with medical treatment: Meta-analysis of the effects of anxiety and depression on patient adherence." *Archives of Internal Medicine 160* (14): 2101–2107. doi:10.1001/archinte.160.14.2101.; Taggart, L. W., J. A. Shaffer, D. Edmondson, et al. 2018. "Posttraumatic stress disorder and nonadherence to medications prescribed for chronic medical conditions: A meta-analysis." *Journal of Psychiatry Research 102*: 102–109. doi:10.1016/j.jpsychires.2018.02.013.
45. Stewart and Rollman 2014.

CHAPTER 3

1. Gleason, L. P., L. X. Deng, A. M. Khan, D. Drajpuch, S. Fuller, J. Ludmir, C. E. Mascio, et al. 2019. "Psychological distress in adults with congenital heart disease: Focus beyond depression." *Cardiology in the Young 29* (2): 185–189. doi:10.1017/S1047951118002068.
2. Callus, E., and G. Pravettoni. 2018. "The role of clinical psychology and peer to peer support in the management of chronic medical conditions— A practical example with adults with congenital heart disease." *Frontiers in Psychology 9* (731). https://www.frontiersin.org/articles/10.3389/fpsyg.2018.00731.
3. McCarty, R. 2016. "The fight-or-flight response: A cornerstone of stress research." In *Stress: Concepts, cognition, emotion, and behavior*, edited by George Fink, 33–37. Academic Press. ISBN 9780128009512, https://doi.org/10.1016/B978-0-12-800951-2.00004-2.
4. Hannibal, K. E., and M. D. Bishop. 2014. "Chronic stress, cortisol dysfunction, and pain: A psychoneuroendocrine rationale for stress management in pain rehabilitation." *Physical Therapy 94* (12): 1816–1825. doi:10.2522/ptj.20130597.

5. Ogden, P., and J. Fisher. 2015. *Sensorimotor psychotherapy: Interventions for trauma and attachment.* (Norton Series on Interpersonal Neurobiology). WW Norton & Company; Levine, P., and M. Kline. 2006. *Trauma through a child's eyes: Awakening the ordinary miracle of healing.* North Atlantic Books, U.S.

6. Porges, S. W. 2011. *The polyvagal theory: Neurophysiological foundations of emotions, attachment, communication, and self-regulation.* W.W. Norton.

7. Porges, S. W. 2021. "Polyvagal theory: A biobehavioral journey to sociality." *Comprehensive Psychoneuroendocrinology* 7: 1–7. https://doi.org/10.1016/j.cpnec.2021.100069.

8. Morton, L. 2018. "Born with a heart condition: The clinical implications of the polyvagal theory." In *Clinical application of the polyvagal theory,* edited by S. W. Porges and D. Dana, 397–418. Norton Professional Books.

9. Hefferon, L., M. Grealy, and N. Mutrie. 2009. "Post-traumatic growth and life-threatening physical illness: A systematic review of the qualitative literature." *British Journal of Health Psychology* 14: 343–378.

10. Roseman, A., L. Morton, and A. H. Kovacs. 2021. "Health anxiety among adults with congenital heart disease." *Current Opinion in Cardiology* 36 (1): 98–104.

11. American Psychiatric Association. 2022. *DSM-5-TR: Diagnostic and statistical manual of mental disorders.* 5th ed., rev. American Psychiatric Association.

12. Levine Peter A. 1997. Waking the Tiger: Healing Trauma: The Innate Capacity to Transform Overwhelming Experiences. Berkeley California: North Atlantic Books.

13. American Psychiatric Association 2022.

14. American Psychiatric Association 2022.

15. Toren, P., and N. Horesh. 2007. "Psychiatric morbidity in adolescents operated in childhood for congenital cyanotic heart disease." *Pediatric Child Health* 43 (10) (October): 662–666.

16. Merikangas, K. R., J. P. He, M. Burstein, S. A. Swanson, S. Avenevoli, L. Cui, C. Benjet, K. Georgiades, and J. Swendsen. 2011. "Lifetime prevalence of mental disorders in U.S. adolescents: Results from the National Comorbidity Survey Replication—Adolescent Supplement (NCS-A)." *Journal of the American Academy of Child and Adolescent Psychiatry* 49 (10): 980–989.

17. Deng, L. X., A. M. Khan, D. Drajpuch, et al. 2016. "Prevalence and correlates of post-traumatic stress disorder in adults with congenital heart disease." *American Journal of Cardiology* 1 (117): 853–857.

18. Helfricht, S., B. Latel, and J. E. Fisher. 2008. "Surgery-related posttraumatic stress disorder in parents of children undergoing cardiopulmonary bypass surgery: A prospective cohort study." *Pediatric Critical Care Medicine* 9 (2): 217–223.

19. Vilchinsky, N., K. Ginzburg, K. Fait, and E. B. Foa. 2017. "Cardiac-disease-induced PTSD (CDI-PTSD): A systematic review." *Clinical Psychology Review* 55: 92–106. https://doi.org/10.1016/j.cpr.2017.04.009.

20. Taggart, L. W., J. A. Shaffer, D. Edmondson, et al. 2018. "Posttraumatic stress disorder and nonadherence to medications prescribed for chronic

medical conditions: A meta-analysis." *Journal of Psychiatric Research 102*: 102–109. doi:10.1016/j.jpsychires.2018.02.013.

21. Edmondson, D., I. M. Kronish, J. A. Falzon, and M. M. Burg. 2013. "Posttraumatic stress disorder and risk for coronary heart disease: A meta-analytic review." *American Heart Journal 166* (5): 806–814. https://doi.org/10.1016/j.ahj.2013.07.031.

22. Zeligman, M., J. A. Bialo, J. A. Brack, and M. A. Kearney. 2017. "Loneliness as moderator between trauma and posttraumatic growth." *Journal of Counseling & Development 95*: 435–444. https://doi.org/10.1002/jcad.12158.

23. Wilson, C. J., F. P. Deane, J. Ciarrochi, and D. Rickwood. 2005. "Measuring help-seeking intentions: Properties of the General Help-Seeking Questionnaire." *Canadian Journal of Counselling 39* (1): 15–28.

24. Morton 2020.

25. Janoff-Bulman, R. 1989. "Assumptive worlds and the stress of traumatic events: Applications of the schema construct." *Social Cognition 7* (2): 113–136. https://doi.org/10.1521/soco.1989.7.2.113.

26. van der Kolk, B. A. 2014. *The body keeps the score: Brain, mind, and body in the healing of trauma.* Viking.

27. Roseman, A., and A. H. Kovacs. 2019. "Anxiety and depression in adults with congenital heart disease: When to suspect and how to refer." *Current Cardiology Reports 21*: 145. https://doi.org/10.1007/s11886-019-1237-2.

28. American Psychiatric Association 2022.

29. American Psychiatric Association. 2022. *DSM-5-TR: Diagnostic and statistical manual of mental disorders.* 5th ed., rev. American Psychiatric Association.

30. American Psychiatric Association 2022.

31. Culpepper, L. 2009. "Generalized anxiety disorder and medical illness." *Journal of Clinical Psychiatry 70* (Suppl. 2): 20–24. doi:10.4088/jcp.s.7002.04. PMID: 19371503.

32. American Psychiatric Association 2022.

33. Hefferon, Grealy, and Mutrie 2009.

CHAPTER 4

1. Kovacs, A. H., A. S. Saidi, E. A. Kuhl, et al. 2009. "Depression and anxiety in adult congenital heart disease: Predicots and prevalence." *International Journal of Cardiology 137*: 158–164.

2. Obama Michelle. 2018. Becoming First ed. New York NY: Crown an imprint of the Crown Publishing Group.

3. Livecchi, T. 2004. "Psychosocial issues affecting adults with congenital heart disease: One patient's perspective." *Nursing Clinics of North America 39* (4): 787–789. doi:10.1016/j.cnur.2004.08.003.

4. White, K. S., C. Pardue, P. Ludbrook, S. Sodhi, A. Esmaeeli, and A. Cedars. 2016. "Cardiac denial and psychological predictors of cardiac care adherence in adults with congenital heart disease." *Behavior Modification 40* (1–2): 29–50.

5. DiMatteo, M. R., H. S. Lepper, and T. W. Croghan. 2000. "Depression is a risk factor for noncompliance with medical treatment: Meta-analysis of the effects of anxiety and depression on patient adherence." *Archives of Internal Medicine 160* (14): 2101–2107. doi:10.1001/archinte.160.14.2101.

6. Wang, J. T., B. Hoffman, and J. A. Blumenthal. 2011. "Management of depressed cardiac patients." *Expert Opinion on Psychopharmacology 12* (1): 85–98.

7. American Psychiatric Association. 2022. *DSM-5-TR: Diagnostic and statistical manual of mental disorders.* 5th ed., rev. American Psychiatric Association.

8. American Psychiatric Association 2022.

9. Pillinger, E. F., I. M. Rodriguez, G. M. Khandaker, C. M. Pariante, and O. D. Howes. 2020. "Inflammatory markers in depression: A meta-analysis of mean differences and variability in 5,166 patients and 5,083 controls." *Brain, Behavior, and Immunity 87*: 901–909. doi:10.1016/j.bbi.2020.02.010.

10. Nutt, D. J. 2008. "Relationship of neurotransmitters to the symptoms of major depressive disorder." *Journal of Clinical Psychiatry 69* (E1): 4–7. https://pubmed.ncbi.nlm.nih.gov/18494537/.

11. Sotile, W., and R. Cantor-Cooke. 2003. *Thriving with heart disease.* Free Press.

12. Miceli, M., and C. Castelfranchi. 2018. "Reconsidering the differences between shame and guilt." *Europe's Journal of Psychology 14* (3): 710–733.

13. Gilbert, P. 2014. "The origins and nature of compassion focused-therapy." *British Journal of Clinical Psychology 53* (1): 6–41.

14. Woolf Virginia Leonard Woolf Vanessa Bell and Hogarth Press. 1930. On Being Ill. London: Printed and published by Leonard & Virginia Woolf at The Hogarth Press.

CHAPTER 5

1. Manjulaa, N., P. Allotey, and A. Hardon. 2019. "Self care interventions to advance health and wellbeing: A conceptual framework to inform normative guidance." *British Medical Journal 365.* doi:10.1136/bmj.l688.

2. Mastin, D. F., J. Bryson, and R. Corwyn. 2006. "Assessment of sleep hygiene using the Sleep Hygiene Index." *Journal of Behavioural Medicine 29*: 223–227.

3. Somerville Heart Foundation. 2020. "Lifestyle issues." Somerville Heart Foundation.

4. British Dietetic Association. 2021. Accessed online at Food and mood | British Dietetic Association (BDA).

5. Netz, Y. 2017. "Is the comparison between exercise and pharmacologic treatment of depression in the clinical practice guideline of the American College of Physicians evidence-based?" *Frontiers in Pharmacology 8* (257).

6. Budts W., G. E. Pieles, J. W. Roos-Hesselink, M. Sanz de la Garza, F. D'Ascenzi, G. Giannakoulas, et al. 2020. Recommendations for participation in competitive sport in adolescent and adult athletes with Congenital Heart Disease (CHD): Position statement of the Sports Cardiology & Exercise Section of the European Association of Preventive Cardiology (EAPC), the European

Society of Cardiology (ESC) Working Group on Adult Congenital Heart Disease and the Sports Cardiology, Physical Activity and Prevention Working Group of the Association for European Paediatric and Congenital Cardiology (AEPC). *European Heart Journal 41* (43): 4191–4199. doi:10.1093/eurheartj/ehaa501. PMID: 32845299.

7. Gatzoulis, M. A., L. Swan, J. Therrien, and G. A. Pantley. 2010. *Adult congenital heart disease: A practical guide.* 2nd ed. Blackwell.

8. Somerville Heart Foundation 2020.

9. Valenza MC, Valenza-Peña G, Torres-Sánchez I, González-Jiménez E, Conde-Valero A, Valenza-Demet G. Effectiveness of controlled breathing techniques on anxiety and depression in hospitalized patients with COPD: a randomized clinical Trial. Respir Care. 2014 Feb;59(2):209-15. doi: 10.4187/respcare.02565. Epub 2013 Jul 23. Erratum in: *Respir Care.* 2016 Nov;61(11):e3. PMID: 23882107.

10. Jacobson, E. (1987). Progressive relaxation. *The American Journal of Psychology,* 100(3/4), 522–537. https://doi.org/10.2307/1422693

11. Chaudhuri, A. 2020. "Is there any effect of progressive muscle relaxation exercise on anxiety and depression of the patient with coronary artery disease?" *International Journal of Pharmaceutical Sciences and Research 8* (5): 3231–3236.

12. Ludwig, D. S., and J. Kabat-Zinn. 2008. "Mindfulness in medicine." *JAMA 300* (11): 1350–1352. doi:10.1001/jama.300.11.1350.

13. Kabat-Zinn, J. 2018. *Meditation is not what you think: Mindfulness and why it is so important.* Hachette Books.

14. Hudson, B. F., P. Ogden, and M. S. Whiteley. 2015. "Randomized controlled trial to compare the effect of simple distraction interventions on pain and anxiety experienced during conscious surgery." *European Journal of Pain 19* (10): 1447–1455.

15. Nash, J. 2014. "Stress and diabetes: The use of 'worry time' as a way of managing stress." *Journal of Diabetes Nursing 18*: 329–332.

16. Butler, G., and T. Hope. 1995. *Manage your mind.* Oxford University Press.

17. Butler and Hope 1995.

CHAPTER 6

1. Frankl, Viktor E. (Viktor Emil), 1905-1997 author. Man's Search for Meaning: an Introduction to Logotherapy. Boston: Beacon Press, 1962.

2. Kira, I. A., N. Arıcı Özcan, H. Schwiekh, et al. 2020. "The compelling dynamics of 'will to exist, live, and survive' on effecting posttraumatic growth upon exposure to adversities: Is it mediated, in part, by emotional regulation, resilience, and spirituality?" *Traumatology 26* (4): 405–419. https://doi.org/10.1037/trm0000263.

3. Hayes, S. C. 2005. *Get out of your mind and into your life: The new acceptance and commitment therapy.* New Harbinger.

4. Dalgleish, T., J. Yiend, S. Schweizer, and B. D. Dunn. 2009. "Ironic effects of emotion suppression when recounting distressing memories." *Emotion 9* (5): 744–749. https://doi.org/10.1037/a0017290.

5. Torre, J. B., and M. D. Lieberman. 2018. "Putting feelings into words: Affect labeling as implicit emotion regulation." *Emotion Review 10* (2): 116–124.

6. Gilbert, P. 2014. "The origins and nature of compassion focused therapy." *British Journal of Clinical Psychology 53* (1): 6–41.

7. Klagsbrun, J., Lennox, S., & Summers, L. (2010). Effect of clearing a space on quality of life in women with breast cancer. *Journal of Body Psychotherapy*, 9, 48–53.

8. Porges, S. W. 2021. "Polyvagal theory: A biobehavioral journey to sociality." *Comprehensive Psychoneuroendocrinology* 7: 1–7. https://doi.org/10.1016/j.cpnec.2021.100069.

9. Porges 2021; Morton, L., N. Cogan, J. Kolacz, M. Nikolic, C. Calderwood, T. Bacon, E. Pathe, and D. Williams. 2022. "A new measure of feeling safe: Developing psychometric properties of the Neuroception of Psychological Safety Scale (NPSS)." *Psychological Trauma: Theory, Research, Practice, and Policy.* https://doi.org/10.1037/tra0001313.

10. Vagnoli L, Bettini A, Amore E, De Masi S, Messeri A. Relaxation-guided imagery reduces perioperative anxiety and pain in children: a randomized study. *Eur J Pediatr.* 2019 Jun;178(6):913–921. doi: 10.1007/s00431-019-03376-x. Epub 2019 Apr 3. PMID: 30944985.

CHAPTER 7

1. Beck, J. S. 2011. *Cognitive behavior therapy: Basics and beyond.* 2nd ed. Guilford Press.

2. Beck 2011.

3. Beck 2011.

4. Beesdo-Baum K, Jenjahn E, Höfler M, Lueken U, Becker ES, Hoyer J. Avoidance, safety behavior, and reassurance seeking in generalized anxiety disorder. *Depress Anxiety.* 2012 Nov;29(11):948-57. doi: 10.1002/da.21955. Epub 2012 May 11. PMID: 22581482.

5. Pim, C., A. V. Straten, and L. Warmerdam. 2007. "Behavioral activation treatments of depression: A meta-analysis." *Clinical Psychology Review 27* (3): 318–326.

6. Mora-Ripoll R. The therapeutic value of laughter in medicine. *Altern Ther Health Med.* 2010 Nov-Dec;16(6):56-64. PMID: 21280463.

CHAPTER 8

1. Wang, J., F. Mann, B. Lloyd-Evans, M. Ruimin, and S. Johnson. 2018. "Associations between loneliness and perceived social support and outcomes of mental health problems: A systematic review." *BMC Psychiatry 18* (156).

2. Holt-Lunstad, J., T. Smith, and J. B. Layton. 2010. "Social relationships and mortality risk: A meta-analytic review." *PLOS Medicine 7* (7) (July).

3. Robert Holden (2011). "Happiness Now!: Timeless Wisdom for Feeling Good Fast", p.72, Hay House, Inc.

4. Fennell, M. J. 1997. "Low self-esteem: A cognitive perspective." *Behavioural and Cognitive Psychotherapy 25*: 1–26.

5. Verstappen, A., D. Pearson, and A. H. Kovacs. 2006. "Adult congenital heart disease: The patient's perspective." *Cardiology Clinics 24*: 515–529.

6. Gilbert, P. 2009. *The compassionate mind.* Robinson.

7. Gilbert 2009.

8. van der Kolk, B. A. 2014. *The body keeps the score: Brain, mind, and body in the healing of trauma.* Viking.

9. Gilbert 2009.

10. Neff, K. D., and C. K. Germer. 2013. "A pilot study and randomized controlled trial of the mindful self-compassion program." *Journal of Clinical Psychology 69*: 28–44.

11. Fredrickson, B., M. Cohn, K. Coffey, J. Pek, and S. Finkel. 2008. "Open hearts build lives: Positive emotions, induced through loving-kindness meditation, build consequential personal resources." *Journal of Personality and Social Psychology 95* (5): 1045–1062.

12. Bowlby, J. 1969. *Attachment and loss.* Basic Books.

13. McWhorter, L., J. Christofferson, T. Neely, A. Hildenbrand, M. Alderfer, A. Randall, and E. Sood. 2022. "Parental post-traumatic stress, overprotective parenting, and emotional and behavioural problems for children with critical congenital heart disease." *Cardiology in the Young 32* (5): 738–745. doi:10.1017/S1047951121002912. Epub 2021 Aug 9. PMID: 34365986; PMCID: PMC8825886.

14. How to deal with sex and heart conditions | BHF, 2021.

15. McCue, K., and R. Bonn. 2011. *How to help children through a parent's serious illness.* 2nd ed. St. Martin's Press.

16. Bion, W. R. 1962. *Learning from experience.* Karnac.

17. Winnicott, D. 1960. "The theory of the parent-child relationship." *International Journal of Psychoanalysis 41*: 585–595.

18. Frankl, Viktor E. (Viktor Emil), 1905–1997 author. Man's Search for Meaning: an Introduction to Logotherapy. Boston :Beacon Press, 1962.

19. Markowitz, J. C., and M. M. Weissman. 2012. "Interpersonal psychotherapy: Past, present and future." *Clinical Psychology and Psychotherapy 19* (2): 99–105.

20. Morton, L. 2011. "Can interpersonal psychotherapy meet the psychological cost of life gifted by medical intervention?" *Counselling Psychology Review 26* (3): 75–86.

CHAPTER 9

1. Congenital Heart Public Health Consortium. 2019. "Know the facts." Retrieved from Congenital Heart Defect Fact Sheets (aap.org); Morton, L. 2020a. "Using psychologically informed care to improve mental health and

wellbeing for people living with a heart condition from birth: A statement paper." *Journal of Health Psychology* 25 (2). https://doi.org/10.1177/135910531 9826354; Salzmann, S., M. Salzmann-Djufri, M. Wilhelm, and F. Euteneuer. 2020. "Psychological preparation for cardiac surgery." *Current Cardiology Reports* 22 (12): 172.

2. Mylotte, D., L. Pilote, R. Ionescu-Ittu, M. Abrahamowicz, P. Khairy, J. Therrien, A. Mackie, and A. Marelli. 2014. "Specialized adult congenital heart disease care: The impact on mortality." *Circulation* 128 (18): 1804–1812.

3. Fernandes, S. M., A. Verstappen, M. Clair, M. Rummell, D. Barber, K. Ackerman, K. Dummer, et al. 2019. "Knowledge of life-long cardiac care by adolescents and young adults with congenital heart disease." *Pediatric Cardiology* 40 (7): 1439–1444. doi:10.1007/s00246-019-02154-8.

4. Stout, K. K., C. J. Daniels, J. A. Aboulhosn, B. Bozkurt, C. S. Broberg, J. M. Colman, S. R. Crumb, et al. 2019. "2018 AHA/ACC guideline for the management of adults with congenital heart disease: Executive summary: A report of the American College of Cardiology/American Heart Association Task Force on Clinical Practice Guidelines." *Circulation* 139 (14): e637–e697. doi:10.1161/CIR.0000000000000602.

5. Assenza, G., E. Krieger, H. Baumgartner, B. Cupido, K. Dimopoulos, C. Louis, A. Lubert, et al. 2021. "AHA/ACC vs ESC guidelines for management of adults with congenital heart disease: JACC guideline comparison." *Journal of the American College of Cardiology* 78 (19). https://doi.org/10.1016/j.jacc.2021.09.010.

6. Van Such, M., R. Lohr, T. Beckman, and J. M. Naessens. 2017. "Extent of diagnostic agreement among medical referrals." *Journal of Evaluation in Clinical Practice* 23 (4): 870–874.

7. Salzmann, S., M. Salzmann-Djufri, M. Wilhelm, and F. Euteneuer. 2020. "Psychological preparation for cardiac surgery." *Current Cardiology Reports* 22 (12): 172.

8. Robertson, J. 1970. *Young children in hospital*. 2nd ed. Tavistock.

9. Hertenstein, M. J., D. Keltner, and B. App. 2006. "Touch communicates distinct emotions." *Emotion* 6: 528–533.

10. Field, T. M., and M. Hernandez-Reif. 2010. "Preterm infant massage therapy research: A review." *Infant Behavioral Development* 33 (2): 115–124.

11. Jefferies, A. L. 2012. "Kangaroo care for the preterm infant and family." *Paediatrics & Child Health* 17 (3): 141–143.

12. Simon-Thomas, E. R., D. J. Keltner, D. Sauter, L. Sinicropi-Yao, and A. Abramson. 2009. "The voice conveys specific emotions: Evidence from vocal burst displays." *Emotion* 9: 838–846.

13. Filippa, M., M. G. Monaci, C. Spagnuolo, P. Serravalle, R. Daniele, and D. Grandjean. 2021. "Maternal speech decreases pain scores and increases oxytocin levels in preterm infants during painful procedures." *Scientific Reports* 11 (17301). https://doi.org/10.1038/s41598-021-96840-4.

14. Huddleston, P. 2012. *Prepare for surgery, heal faster: A guide of mind-body techniques.* 4th ed. Angel River Press.

15. Halpin, L., A. Speir, P. CapoBianco, and S. Barnett. 2002. "Guided imagery in cardiac surgery." *Outcomes Management 6* (3): 132–137.

16. Huddleston 2012.

17. Huddleston 2012.

18. British Congenital Cardiac Association. 2020. "BCCA COVID-19 guidance for vulnerable groups with congenital heart disease." https://www.bcca-uk. org/pages/news_box.asp?NewsID=19495710

19. Cousino, M. K., S. K. Pasquali, J. C. Romano, M. D. Norris, S. Yu, G. Reichle, R. Lowery, S. Viers, and K. R. Schumacher. 2021. "Impact of the COVID-19 pandemic on CHD care and emotional wellbeing." *Cardiology in the Young 31* (5): 822–828. https://doi.org/10.1017/S1047951120004758.

20. Morton, L., C. Calderwood, N. Cogan, C. Murphy, E. Nix, and J. Kolacz. 2022. "An exploration of psychological trauma and positive adaptation in adults with congenital heart disease during the COVID-19 pandemic." *Patient Experience Journal 9* (1): 82–94. doi:10.35680/2372-0247.1638.

21. Morton, Calderwood, Cogan, Murphy, Nix, and Kolacz 2022.

22. Personal interview with Tracy Livecchi, September 2021.

23. Personal interview with Tracy Livecchi, September 2021.

24. A. Leibold, E. Eichler, S. Chung, et al. 2021. "Pain in adults with congenital heart disease—An international perspective." *International Journal of Cardiology Congenital Heart Disease 5*: 100200.

CHAPTER 10

1. Frankl, Viktor E. (Viktor Emil), 1905-1997 author. Man's Search for Meaning: an Introduction to Logotherapy. Boston: Beacon Press, 1962.

2. Equality Act, 2010, UK Government. https://www.gov.uk/guidance/equality-act-2010-guidance

3. WHO, 2022 – retrieval info Disability and health (who.int) https://www.who.int/news-room/fact-sheets/detail/disability-and-health

4. Bogart, K. R., E. M. Lund, and A. Rottenstein. 2018. "Disability pride protects self-esteem through the rejection identification model." *Rehabilitation Psychology 63* (1): 155–159. https://doi.org/10.1037/rep0000166.

5. Rowe, M. 2015. *Citizenship and mental health.* Oxford University Press.

6. Bogart, K., A. Rottenstein, E. M. Lund, and L. Bouchard. 2017. "Who self-identifies as disabled? An examination of impairment and contextual predictors." *Rehabilitation Psychology 62* (4): 553–562. https://doi.org/10.1037/rep0000132; Bogart, Lund, and Rottenstein 2018.

7. Oliver 2013.

8. Oliver M. 2013. "The social model of disability: thirty years on." *Disability & Society 28*: 7, 1024–1026. doi:10.1080/09687599.2013.818773.

9. Steinert, C., T. Steinert, E. Flammer, and S. Jaeger. 2016. "Impact of the UN Convention on the Rights of Persons with Disabilities (UN-CRPD) on mental health care research—A systematic review." *BMC Psychiatry 16* (166). https://doi.org/10.1186/s12888-016-0862-1.
10. Americans with Disabilities Act, 1990. https://adata.org/factsheet/ADA-overview
11. Zomer, A. C., I. Vaartjes, C. S. Uiterwaal, E. T. van der Velde, G. J. Sieswerda, E. M. Wajon, K. Plomp, et al. 2012. "Social burden and lifestyle in adults with congenital heart disease." *American Journal of Cardiology 109* (11): 1657–1663. https://doi.org/10.1016/j.amjcard.2012.01.397.
12. Gong, C. L., H. Zhao, Y. Wei, et al. 2020. "Lifetime burden of adult congenital heart disease in the USA using a microsimulation model." *Pediatric Cardiology* https:// doi.org/10.1007/s00246-020-02409-9.
13. Morton, L. 2020b. "Ableism in psychology: Every choice has been dictated by my health condition." *The Psychologist 33* (6).
14. Equality Act 2010.
15. Birkeland Nielsen, M., J. Shahid Emberland, and S. Knardahl. 2017. "Workplace bullying as a predictor of disability retirement: A prospective registry study of Norwegian employees." *Journal of Occupational and Environmental Medicine 59* (7): 609–614. doi:10.1097/JOM.0000000000001026.
16. Morton 2020b.
17. Meentken, M., M. van der Mheen, I. M. van Beynum, E. M. Utens, et al. 2021. "Long-term effectiveness of eye movement desensitization and reprocessing in children and adolescents with medically related subthreshold post-traumatic stress disorder: A randomized controlled trial." *European Journal of Cardiovascular Nursing 20* (4).
18. Assenzsa, G. E., K. Dimopoulos, W. Budts, A. Donti, K. E. Economy, G. D. Gargiulo, M. Gatzoulis, and M. Landzberg. 2021. Online ahead of print. Management of acute cardiovascular complications in pregnancy. *European Heart Journal.* doi:10.1093/eurheartj/ehab546; Scottish Obstetric Cardiac Network (SOCN). 2021. "Do you have a heart condition? Are you pregnant? Ask for advice." https://www.socn.scot.nhs.uk/
19. Bhatt, A., E. Foster, K. Kuehl, J. Alpert, S. Brabeck, S. Crumb, W. Davidson Jr., et al. 2015. "Congenital heart disease in the older adult." *Circulation 131* (21): 1884–1931. https://www.ahajournals.org/doi/10.1161/CIR.0000000000000204.
20. Small, J. A., D. Karlin, C. Jain, J. M. Steiner, and L. C. Reardon. 2021. "Advance care planning in adult congenital heart disease: Unique approaches for a unique population." *International Journal of Cardiology Congenital Heart Disease 5.* https://doi.org/10.1016/j.ijcchd.2021.100203.
21. Rogers, C. R. 1. (1961). On becoming a person: a therapist's view of psychotherapy. Boston: Houghton Mifflin.
22. Wilson, K. G., and A. R. Murrell. 2004. "Values work in acceptance and commitment therapy: Setting a course for behavioral treatment." In *Mindfulness*

and acceptance: Expanding the cognitive-behavioral tradition, edited by S. C. Hayes, V. M. Follette, and M. M. Linehan, 120–151. Guilford Press.

23. Doran, G. T. 1981. "There's a S.M.A.R.T. way to write management's goals and objectives." *Management Review 70* (11): 35–36.

CHAPTER 11

1. Angelou Maya. 2008. Letter to My Daughter. 1st ed. New York: Random House.
2. Calhoun, L. G., and R. G. Tedeschi. 2004. "The foundations of posttraumatic growth: New considerations." *Psychological Inquiry 15* (1): 93–102.
3. Albrecht, G. L., and P. L. Devlieger. 1999. "The disability paradox: High quality of life against all odds." *Social Science & Medicine 48* (8): 977–988.
4. Calhoun and Tedeschi 2004.
5. Morton, L., C. Calderwood, N. Cogan, C. Murphy, E. Nix, and J. Kolacz. 2022. "An exploration of psychological trauma and positive adaptation in adults with congenital heart disease during the COVID-19 pandemic." *Patient Experience Journal 9* (1): 82–94. doi:10.35680/2372-0247.1638.
6. Collier, L. 2016. "Growth after trauma." *Monitor on Psychology 47* (10).
7. Cyrulnik, B. 2011. *Resilience: How your inner strength can set you free.* Penguin.
8. Jung, C. G., H. Read, M. Forham, G. Alder, and R. F. C. Hull. 1966. *The collected works of C.G. Jung.* Princeton University Press.
9. Tedeschi, R. G., J. Shakespear-Finch, J. Taku, and L. G. Calhoun. 2018. *Posttraumatic growth: Theory, research, and applications.* Routledge.
10. Morton, Calderwood, Cogan, Murphy, Nix, and Kolacz 2022.
11. Greater Good Science Center, UC Berkeley. 2018. "The science of gratitude." https://ggsc.berkeley.edu/; Wong, J., J. Owen, N. Gabana, J. Brown, S. McInnis, P. Toth, and L. Gilman. 2016. "Does gratitude writing improve the mental health of psychotherapy clients? Evidence from a randomized controlled trial." *Psychotherapy Research 28* (2): 1–11.
12. Greater Good Science Center, UC Berkeley 2018.
13. Lyubomirsky, S. 2007. *The how of happiness.* Penguin.

CHAPTER 12

1. Ntiloudi, D., M. A. Gatzoulis, A. Alexandra, H. Karvounis, and G. Giannakoulas. 2021. "Adult congenital heart disease: Looking back, moving forward." *International Journal of Cardiology Congenital Heart Disease 2*: 100076. ISSN 2666-6685, https://doi.org/10.1016/j.ijcchd.2020.100076.
2. Morton, L. 2020a. "Using psychologically informed care to improve mental health & wellbeing for people living with a heart condition from birth: A statement paper." *Journal of Health Psychology 25* (2). https://doi.org/10.1177/1359105319826354.

3. Guggenbühl-Craig, A. 1998. *Power in the helping professions*. Springer.

4. Bray, L., K. Ford, and A. Dickenson. 2018. "A qualitative study of health professionals' views on the holding of children for clinical procedures: Constructing a balanced approach." *Journal of Child Health Care* 22 (3): 1–16; Morton, L., N. Cogan, S. Kornfält, Z. Porter, and E. Georgiadis. 2020d. "Baring all: The impact of the hospital gown on patient wellbeing." *British Journal of Health Psychology* 25 (3). doi.org/10.1111/bjhp.12416.

5. Morton, L., N. Cogan, J. Kolacz, M. Nikolic, C. Calderwood, T. Bacon, E. Pathe, and D. Williams. 2022. "A new measure of feeling safe: Developing psychometric properties of the Neuroception of Psychological Safety Scale (NPSS)." *Psychological Trauma: Theory, Research, Practice, and Policy*. https://doi.org/10.1037/tra0001313.

6. Gilbert, P. 2014. "The origins and nature of compassion focused therapy." *British Journal of Clinical Psychology* 53 (1): 6–41.

7. Mollon, D. 2014. "Feeling safe during an inpatient hospitalization: A concept analysis." *Journal of Advanced Nursing* 70 (8): 1727–1737.

8. Morton 2020a.

9. Field, T. M., and M. Hernandez-Reif. 2010. "Preterm infant massage therapy research: A review." *Infant Behavioral Development* 33 (2): 115–124.

10. Čartolovni, A., M. Stolt, and R. Suhonen. 2021. "Moral injury in healthcare professionals: A scoping review and discussion." *Nursing Ethics* 11. doi:10.1177/0969733020966776.

11. Hertenstein, M. J., D. Keltner, and B. App. 2006. "Touch communicates distinct emotions." *Emotion* 6: 528–533.

12. Jefferies, A. L. 2012. "Kangaroo care for the preterm infant and family." *Paediatrics & Child Health* 17 (3): 141–143.

13. Field and Hernandez-Reif 2010.

14. Simon-Thomas, E. R., D. J. Keltner, D. Sauter, L. Sinicropi-Yao, and A. Abramson. 2009. "The voice conveys specific emotions: Evidence from vocal burst displays." *Emotion* 9: 838–846.

15. Filippa, M., M. G. Monaci, C. Spagnuolo, P. Serravalle, R. Daniele, and D. Grandjean. 2021. "Maternal speech decreases pain scores and increases oxytocin levels in preterm infants during painful procedures." *Scientific Reports* 11 (17301). https://doi.org/10.1038/s41598-021-96840-4.

16. Robertson, J. 1970. *Young children in hospital*. 2nd ed. Tavistock.

17. Morton, L. 2019. "NHS needs to learn how people living with serious heart disease feel about it." *The Scotsman*, October.

18. Meentken, M. G., I. M. van Beyman, J. S. Legerstee, et al. 2017. "Medically related post-traumatic stress in children and adolescents with congenital heart defects." *Frontiers in Paediatrics* 5 (20).

19. Deng, L. X., A. M. Khan, D. Drajpuch, et al. 2016. "Prevalence and correlates of post-traumatic stress disorder in adults with congenital heart disease." *American Journal of Cardiology* 1 (117): 853–857.

20. Vilchinsky, N., K. Ginzburg, K. Fait, and E. B. Foa. 2017. "Cardiac-disease-induced PTSD (CDI-PTSD): A systematic review." *Clinical Psychology Review* 55: 92–106. https://doi.org/10.1016/j.cpr.2017.04.009.

21. Vilchinsky, Ginzburg, Fait, and Foa 2017.

22. Roseman, A., L. Morton, and A. H. Kovacs. 2021. "Health anxiety among adults with congenital heart disease." *Current Opinion in Cardiology 36* (1): 98–104.

23. Detsky, A. S., & Krumholz, H. M. (2014). Reducing the trauma of hospitalization. *JAMA*, 311(21), 2169–2170.

24. Morton, L., N. Cogan, S. Kornfält, Z. Porter, and E. Georgiadis. 2020d. "Baring all: The impact of the hospital gown on patient wellbeing." *British Journal of Health Psychology 25* (3). doi.org/10.1111/bjhp.12416.

25. Morton, L. 2021a. "Waiting patiently: Healthcare systems need to better address waiting across the patient journey to support health, wellbeing, recovery, and trust." *British Medical Journal* (April). https://blogs.bmj.com/bmj/2021/04/15/liza-morton-waiting-patiently/.

26. Morton 2020a.

27. Callus, E., and G. Pravettoni. 2018. "The role of clinical psychology and peer to peer support in the management of chronic medical conditions—A practical example with adults with congenital heart disease." *Frontiers in Psychology 9* (731). doi:10.3389/fpsyg.2018.00731.

28. Ntiloudi, Gatzoulis, Alexandra, Karvounis, and Giannakoulas 2021.

29. Roseman, A., and A. H. Kovacs. 2019. "Anxiety and depression in adults with congenital heart disease: When to suspect and how to refer." *Current Cardiology Reports* 21: 145. https://doi.org/10.1007/s11886-019-1237-2

30. Morton 2020a; Ogden, P., and J. Fisher. 2015. *Sensorimotor psychotherapy: Interventions for trauma and attachment.* WW Norton & Company; Porges, S. W. 2011. *The polyvagal theory: Neurophysiological foundations of emotions, attachment, communication, and self-regulation.* W.W. Norton.

31. Gilbert 2014.

About the Authors

This book was a labor of love, co-created by two friends, each living with a CHC dependent on pioneering treatment from birth.

Tracy Livecchi, LCSW, is a Clinical Social Worker in Private Practice and the Mental Health Consultant to the Adult Congenital Heart Association's Peer Mentorship Program. Tracy was born with a complicated CHC which has made it necessary for her to have several cardiac surgeries and hospitalizations throughout her life. She feels fortunate to be able to combine her lived experience with a meaningful profession that she loves. She is passionate about improving access to mental health care for all, with a special focus on individuals living with serious and chronic illness. Tracy lives in Connecticut with her husband and two daughters. Follow Tracy on Twitter or Instagram @TracyLivecchi, or find out more at www.tracylivecchi.com.

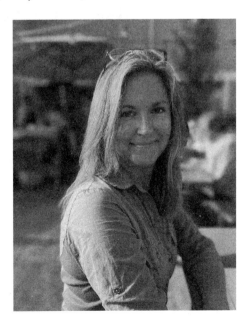

Liza Morton, PhD, C.Psychol, is a Registered Counseling Psychologist in Private Practice and a Lecturer in Applied Psychology at Glasgow Caledonian University. As a health advocate for over ten years, Liza voluntarily sits on the management board of The UK's Somerville Heart Foundation successfully campaigning for Scottish CHD healthcare standards and improved psychological support. Born with complete heart block and a hole in her heart, in a world first at the time, Liza was fitted with her first cardiac pacemaker at just 11 days old in 1978. Dependent on pioneering medical treatment ever since she has faced countless cardiac surgeries, treatments, and hospitalizations. Liza is passionate about promoting what she terms Psychologically Informed Medicine to improve well-being and recovery for people living with lifelong medical conditions. This approach is grounded in her clinical work, research and advocacy and she publishes and presents widely. She lives in Scotland with her husband Craig, their son Dylan and Scottish Terrier Lass. Follow Liza on Twitter or Instagram @ drlizamorton, or find out more at www.drlizamorton.com, photo credit: Colin McPherson.

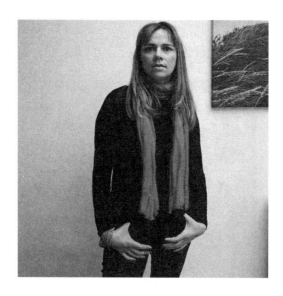

Index

For the benefit of digital users, indexed terms that span two pages (e.g., 52–53) may, on occasion, appear on only one of those pages.

Tables and figures are indicated by *t* and *f* following the page number.

power of attorney, 188
pre-conception counseling, 184
pregnancy, 26–27, 183–86
    CHCs developing in, 6–8
    risk factors for, 184–86
pre-surgery/pre-procedure, 155–57
pride, with disability, 173–76
priorities, 168–70, 194
procedures. *See* medical procedures
prognosis, 36
progressive muscle relaxation, 85
prophylaxis antibiotics, 81
psychiatric illness, 36–37
psychologically informed medicine,
    206–7
psychological safety, 100–1
    compassionate–reflective practice,
    207–9
    guided visualization, 100–1
psychologist, 149*f*
Psychology Today website, 181
PTSD. *See* posttraumatic stress disorder
    (PTSD)
pulmonary arteriovenous aneurysm
    fistula or malformation, 7*t*
pulmonary hypertension, 184
pulmonary stenosis, 7*t*

quality of life, 22–23, 116, 192

radical acceptance, 92
reassurance seeking, 105–6, 113–14
recovery
    longer term recovery, 160–61
    post-surgery recovery, 159–60
relationships, 119–43
    building team exercise, 142–43
    dating, 131
    dealing with unhelpful positivity,
    141–42
    developing healthy communication
    and boundaries, 139–41
    developing independence, 127
    friends and relatives, 136–39
    intimate relationships, 132–33
    loss of parent or caregiver, 129–30
    parenting, 133–34
    with parents or caregivers, 127–29
    parents talking to children about
    CHC, 134–36

posttraumatic growth and, 195
replacing self-criticism with self-
    compassion, 122–27
with yourself, 119–22
relaxation
    progressive muscle relaxation, 85
    scheduling pleasant and relaxing
    events, 81–82
    techniques, 83–84
resentment, 66–69, 141
resilience
    building, 82–83
    posttraumatic growth and, 192–93
rights, disability, 176–78
    patient rights, 177
    United Nations Convention on the
    Rights of Persons with Disabilities
    (UN-CRPD), 177–78
risk-taking behaviors, 117
Ross, Donald, 4
Ross procedure, 4
Rubella, 8
rules for living, 108–11
    tips for challenging, 110–11
    unhelpful beliefs, 110

SAD (seasonal affect disorder), 66
sadness, 92*t*
safety
    abusive or toxic relationships, 137–39
    behaviors, 113–14
    compassionate–reflective practice,
    207–9
    increase feelings of psychological
    safety, 100–1
    safety-seeking behaviors, 48–49
saunas, 81
scarring, 31–32, 131, 156
SDI (socio-demographic index), 23–24
seasonal affect disorder (SAD), 66
second opinions, 148
self-care, 154–61
    building resilience, 82–83
    controlled breathing, 84
    coping during surgery and medical
    procedures, 154–55
    diet and exercise, 77–80
    distraction, 87–88
    Jacobson's progressive muscle
    relaxation, 85